7 DAY Fat Burning

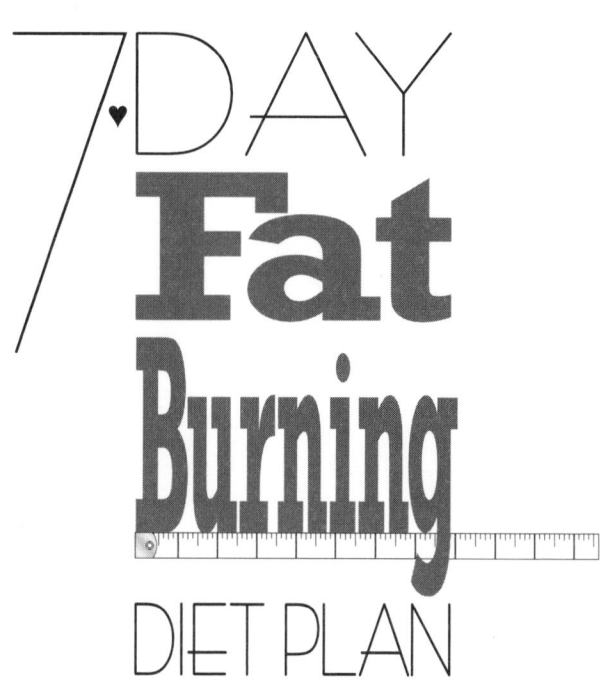

DIET PLAN

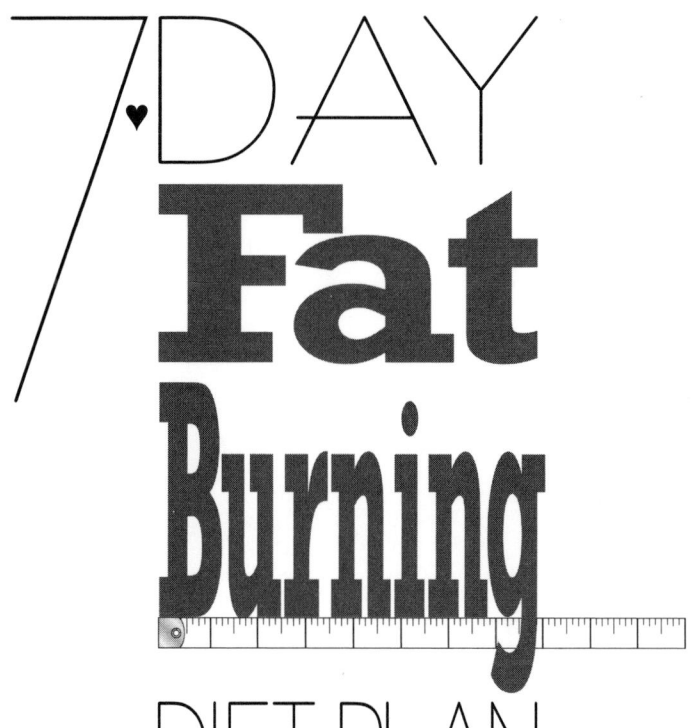

7 DAY Fat Burning DIET PLAN

Change Your Eating Habits for Life

—— CATHERINE ATKINSON ——

foulsham

LONDON • NEW YORK • TORONTO • SYDNEY

foulsham

The Publishing House, Bennetts Close,
Cippenham, Slough, Berks, SL1 5AP, England

ISBN 0-572-02565-3

Printed in Great Britain by St. Edmundsbury Press, Bury St. Edmunds, Suffolk.

CONTENTS

INTRODUCTION

Almost half the adult population in the Western world is overweight, and one in three women and one in five men are on a 'diet' at any time – yet most fail to lose the desired weight or simply put it all back on within a few months. Not only that, but heart disease is rampant, and one of the main culprits is our fat-heavy diet.

Cheer up! Whether you're slimming for the first or fiftieth time, or whether you have been advised by your doctor or dietician to reduce your fat intake and follow a fat-burning diet, this carefully structured plan offers you an easy introduction to a way of eating that will result in permanent weight loss because it will offer your body the right nutrients in the right quantities and balance. Forget about food fads and crash diets – they don't work. You have to change the way you eat.

The good news is just a glance through the inventive and inspiring recipes in this book will persuade you that it will be a change for the better in every respect. With over 100 stunning recipes, you can eat well and wisely without denying yourself the foods you love. Simply use the seven-day plan to get you started – and you need never look back.

WHAT IS THE FAT-BURNING DIET?

There's no doubt that very low-calorie diets can result in rapid weight loss, but the idea that the body can lose up to 3 kg/7 lb of fat in a week is ridiculous – maximum fat loss is unlikely to be more than 900 g/2 lb – any further weight loss shown on the scales will just mean that your body is retaining less water. Another big problem with diets below 1,000 calories a day is that they trigger the body's defence mechanisms so that it treats this reduction of food as a threat and may slow its metabolic rate (the rate at which you burn up calories) by as much as 45 per cent. This means that if you return to your old style of eating, you are likely to regain weight rapidly, not to mention the fact that the old habits were responsible for your weight or health problems in the first place, so you may end up back where you started.

It's not just how much or little food that makes the difference to your weight, but the kind of food you eat.

Most of us eat much more saturated fat and sugar and much less starch (complex carbohydrates) than we should. The average person gets about 40 per cent of their daily calories from fat, about 12 per cent from protein and 48 per cent from carbohydrates. For a healthy diet, no more than 30 per cent of the calories in your diet should come from fat, around 15 per cent from protein and at least 55 per cent (and preferably much more) from carbohydrates, ideally complex carbohydrates.

The fat-burning diet combines carbohydrates, proteins and fats in these correct proportions to maximise the body's fat-burning potential and also ensures a sufficiently high calorie intake to avoid a drop in metabolic rate. In that way, it ensures a steady weight loss for those who are overweight, and provides a balanced diet to maintain good health.

A HEALTHY BALANCE

For any good diet, it is essential to ensure that you have a balanced intake of all the essential food types. This chapter will guide you towards a healthy, balanced diet, either to help you lose weight, or to help you keep your weight at an optimum level and improve your overall health.

CARBOHYDRATES

Not so long ago, all carbohydrates were considered 'fattening' and were the first items to be cut from a slimming diet. We now know that this was wrong. There are two forms of carbohydrate – sugars (simple carbohydrates) and starches (complex carbohydrates); both contain about 4 calories per gram but they are quite different in the way they work in your body.

When the level of glucose in your bloodstream drops, you feel hungry. If you eat simple carbohydrates – such as sugar, honey, syrup, treacle, glucose or fructose – these blood sugar levels rapidly increase and you get a surge in energy, but this is followed by a slump in energy to a level even lower than the original low that caused the craving, so you feel hungry again. So not only do simple carbohydrates create this glucose roller-coaster which plays havoc with the appetite, they contain only 'empty' calories: lots of calories but no nutritional value.

The Glycaemic Index (GI) is a measure of how quickly a food releases its energy and raises your blood sugar level: the higher the GI, the higher the food raises your blood sugar level. A slow increase in blood sugar is healthier than a sudden rise. Foods with a low GI can therefore help control the appetite.

What we need to do, therefore, is to eat foods which help to maintain a steady level of glucose in the bloodstream and provide the essential energy and nutrients the body needs. These foods are the complex carbohydrates – starchy foods such as grains, potatoes and pasta, which are the ideal fat-burning foods. They release energy slowly as they are digested and keep hunger at bay for longer. They also contain the B group of vitamins which help to release energy and combat stress. Meals high in complex carbohydrates raise the metabolic rate of overweight people more than meals that have an identical number of calories but contain mainly proteins and fats. Many athletes improve their endurance by 'carbohydrate loading' before a race. The body converts the starches into glucose in the bloodstream, which gives instant energy, and into glycogen, which provides stored energy. Of all the starchy staples, pasta has the lowest GI score, closely followed by vegetables, rice and bulgar (cracked) wheat.

For a healthy diet, you should therefore reduce your sugar intake and include plenty of starches from a variety of sources.

EASY WAYS TO CUT DOWN ON SUGAR

There's no need to cut out high-sugar foods altogether, but do try to cut down gradually so that eventually you get used to eating less sugar. Try these simple ways of reducing your sugar intake.

- If you add sugar to tea and coffee or breakfast cereals, add a little less every day until you can manage without, or use artificial sweeteners if you must.
- Buy low-calorie mixers and drinks or, better still, mineral or soda water, which can also be used to dilute white wine and fruit juices.
- Replace sweetened fruit yoghurts with low-fat, low-sugar, real fruit varieties, and instead of canned fruits in syrup buy fruits in natural juices.
- Read labels carefully and buy items like tomato ketchup (catsup) and baked beans without added sugar. The same applies to peanut butter, but eat it in small quantities; it is very high in calories.
- Moderate your alcohol intake (see also page 12).

FAT

Fat can be good for you! We tend to think that all fat is bad for our health, but we need some types of fat to stay healthy.

It's useful to know a bit about different types of fat before changing the way we eat. Fats are made up of building blocks of fatty acids and glycerol. There are three types of fatty acids: saturated, polyunsaturated and monounsaturated. Almost all foods that contain fat have a mixture of all three.

Saturated fats are the ones we should really cut down on. They are mainly found in food of animal origin – meat and dairy products such as butter and lard (shortening). A few margarines and oils are made by changing some of the unsaturated fatty acids to saturated ones; these are labelled 'hydrogenated vegetable oil' and should be avoided. Too much fat, and saturated fat in particular, can raise the level of harmful blood cholesterol and increase the risk of heart disease and other illnesses. The body finds it hard to process the fatty acid into energy, and simply stores it as fat, so you should eat as little saturated fat as possible.

Monounsaturated fats are found in foods such as olive oil, some nuts, oily fish and avocado pears. They may help lower the level of blood cholesterol, which could explain why there is such a low incidence of heart disease in Mediterranean countries, but also a high level of obesity in later life. Our bodies can make both saturated and monounsaturated fatty acids, so we do not have to eat them.

Polyunsaturated fats are the ones we need to include in our diet, which is why these are known as **essential fatty acids**. There are two types: omega-6, which can be found in sunflower, sesame, walnut and wheatgerm oils and seeds; and omega-3, from soya and rapeseed oil, walnuts and oily fish such as mackerel and salmon. It's worth reading labels, which will tell you the saturated, monunsaturated and polyunsaturated fat content of foods.

The amount of fat your body actually needs is tiny: a mere teaspoon of polyunsaturated oil daily is enough. Remember that fat contains a massive 9 calories per gram, so cut out as much as you can from your diet and aim to eat no more than 20 to 30 per cent of calories from fat each day if you want to trim your waistline.

TOP FAT-BURNING FOODS

These fat-burning foods are high in complex carbohydrates and low in fat. Eat more of them!

Apples	Peas
Apricots	Pears
Asparagus	Peaches and nectarines
Bananas	Pineapple
Broccoli	Plums
Cabbage	Potatoes
Citrus fruit	Pulses, fresh, canned
Grains: barley, bulgar	and dried
(cracked) wheat,	Root vegetables
couscous, oats, rice	Sweetcorn (corn)
Melon	Tomatoes
Pasta	

EASY WAYS TO CUT DOWN ON FAT

Most of us eat about 100 g/4 oz of fat daily. Yet all we need is 10 g/scant ½ oz; that's the amount in a single rasher (slice) of bacon or a teaspoon of butter or margarine. There are lots of simple ways to reduce your fat intake.

- Use skimmed milk instead of whole milk – there's the same amount of fat in 200 ml/7 fl oz/scant 1 cup of skimmed milk as in 5 ml/1 tsp of whole milk. If you find the switch difficult, try semi-skimmed instead.
- Replace full-fat cheese with reduced-fat cheeses or try medium-fat cheeses such as Edam, Feta, Mozzarella and Brie.
- Invest in a heavy-based, non-stick frying pan (skillet), so you can cook with little or no added fat and use non-stick cookware or line tins (pans) with non-stick baking parchment.
- Dry-fry fatty foods, such as minced (ground) meat and bacon, allowing them to cook in their own fat rather than adding extra. Strain off excess fat or blot it up with kitchen paper (paper towels).
- Buy lean cuts of meat and choose low-fat meats like skinless turkey or chicken. Trim meat of all visible fat. Skim surface fat from casseroles (the easiest way is to allow it to cool so that the fat rises and sets on the top).
- Grill (broil), steam, microwave or bake rather than fry (sauté), and roast meat on a rack over a roasting tin so that the fat can drain off.
- Get into the habit of eating bread without butter or spread. When making sandwiches, add salad filling to keep them moist.

PROTEIN

A healthy diet must include protein. As well as being vital for tissue growth and repair, it is used to make antibodies and hormones. The building blocks in protein are called **amino acids**. There are 25 types, but only eight are essential – the others can be made from these. The best-quality protein foods in terms of amino acid balance include animal sources such as beef, lamb, pork, poultry, fish, eggs, cheese and milk. These are all high in essential amino acids, but unfortunately some are also high in saturated fat and so should be eaten with a high proportion of starchy, fat-burning carbohydrate foods.

Most of us eat at least twice as much animal protein as we need, so try to eat meat-free main meals at least twice a week. Grains, nuts, pulses (dried peas, beans and lentils) and foods such as soya, tofu and Quorn are also good sources of protein. Have two or three small portions of protein a day – if you eat a varied diet, you can be sure you're getting enough!

VITAMINS AND MINERALS

Although needed in much smaller amounts than protein, carbohydrate or fat, vitamins and minerals are vital for general health and well-being. They are required to produce energy, balance hormones and boost the immune system; in fact, almost every body process relies on them. They are found in many foods but the best sources are fruit and vegetables. Eat at least five portions a day, including dark green, leafy vegetables.

FIBRE

Fibre is made up of indigestible carbohydrates and is found in large quantities in any diet that is high in fruit, vegetables, pulses and whole grains. We should all eat more fibre. It passes through the body, absorbing water and waste products, and helps move the food through the gut. Some kinds, such as those found in oats, are 'soluble' fibre and slow down the absorption of carbohydrates, so helping to keep blood sugar levels balanced.

ALCOHOL

Most of us enjoy a drink now and then, especially at social events like parties, and the occasional drink won't ruin your diet. Remember, though, that alcohol is in itself high in calories, and also that after a few drinks your resolve to stick to your diet may weaken.

The healthiest way is to enjoy small amounts of alcohol with food. In fact, it's believed that a daily glass of red wine may even be of benefit as it can help reduce harmful cholesterol.

EXERCISE

Exercise plays an important part in weight loss and health. Moderate, regular exercise keeps your metabolic rate high, which helps to burn off body fat. It also gives your heart and muscles a good work-out and encourages your body to burn fat rather than using carbohydrate stores or muscle.

You don't have to become a fitness freak to take advantage of the effects of exercise. To maximise weight loss, aerobic activities like brisk walking, swimming and cycling are all suitable. Try to find time for three 30-minute sessions a week to give your metabolism a boost.

7-DAY FAT-BURNING MENU PLAN

In this chapter, you'll find a seven-day menu plan to get you started on the fat-burning diet. It's intended as a guide to introduce you to a new way of healthy eating. You can follow it exactly, or you can start to customise it from day one! All the recipes show the proportions of carbohydrates, protein and fat and are also calorie counted. If you are a woman and have less than 13 kg/2 stone to lose, aim to eat around 1,200 calories daily. If you are a man, or have more than 13 kg/2 stone to lose, stick to around 1,500 calories daily. At this level you should lose weight steadily. Once you get a feel for the diet, you can stop counting calories.

Allow yourself one breakfast (you don't have to stick to those suggested here – see page 28 for alternatives), one light meal, one main meal and one dessert daily. Add a snack only if your calorie allowance permits and if you're really hungry; they're not compulsory! If you prefer, you can have a snack instead of dessert. If you make one of the bakes in the snack section, divide it into portions and freeze the extras out of temptation's way. Drink plenty of water throughout the day. You can also have up to 250 ml/8 fl oz/1 cup skimmed milk for tea and coffee, which will add an extra 70 calories. If you're on a 1,500 calorie diet, you can choose an extra snack or two, or a meal accompaniment from the Vegetables and Salads chapter.

MONDAY

		Calories
Breakfast	1 Blueberry Breakfast Bun (page 19)	135
Light meal	Red Bean Burritos (page 48)	290
Main meal	Chicken and Wild Mushroom Lasagne (page 60)	510
Dessert	Frozen Vanilla Yoghurt (page 132)	110
Snack	1 Fruit and Nut Crunch Bar (page 149)	100
	250 ml/8 fl oz/1 cup skimmed milk for tea and coffee	70
Total		1,215

TUESDAY

		Calories
Breakfast	Fresh Apple and Hazelnut Muesli (page 18)	130
Light meal	Pernod-glazed Prawn and Bacon Kebabs (page 36)	340
Main meal	Beef with Red Peppers in Paprika Sauce (page 78)	460
Dessert	Grilled Papaya with Ginger (page 136)	60
Snack	Bruschetta with Soft Goats' Cheese, Rocket and Sun-dried Tomato (page 142)	195
	250 ml/8 fl oz/1 cup skimmed milk for tea and coffee	70
Total		1,255

WEDNESDAY

		Calories
Breakfast	Fruity Wheatgerm Shake (page 21)	230
Light meal	Roasted Red Pepper Soup with Garlic Croûtons (page 30)	230
Main meal	Lamb Cutlets with Hot Apricot Tabbouleh (page 66)	305
Dessert	Dark Chocolate Soufflé (page 134)	180
Snack	Three-bean Tahini Dip with Breadsticks and Crudités (page 148)	235
	250 ml/8 fl oz/1 cup skimmed milk for tea and coffee	70
Total		1,250

THURSDAY

		Calories
Breakfast	Creamed Porridge with Peaches (page 23)	280
Light meal	Saffron and Coriander Steamed Mussels (page 37)	300
Main meal	Duck Satay with Aromatic Rice (page 64)	375
Dessert	Strawberry and Lemon Filo Tartlet (page 133)	70
Snack	Carrot and Courgette Cake with Cream Cheese Frosting (page 154)	115
	250 ml/8 fl oz/1 cup skimmed milk for tea and coffee	70
Total		1,210

FRIDAY

		Calories
Breakfast	Rosti with Baked Tomatoes and Crisp Bacon Curls (page 24)	200
Light meal	Garlic Mushrooms and Dill Dip (page 46)	235
Main meal	Plaice and Vegetable Parcels (page 86)	285
Dessert	Sparkling Orange Jellies with Minted Crème Fraîche (page 126)	200
Snack	Date and Oat Slice (page 146)	230
	250 ml/8 fl oz/1 cup skimmed milk for tea and coffee	70
Total		1,220

SATURDAY

		Calories
Breakfast	Kidney, Bacon and Mushroom Kebabs (page 26)	290
	100 ml/3½ fl oz/scant ½ cup unsweetened orange juice	35
Light meal	Smoked Trout Mousse with Melba Toast (page 40)	195
Main meal	Spaghetti Leonardo (page 93)	340
	Large green side salad without dressing	30
Dessert	Peach Yoghurt Brûlée (page 127)	125
Snack	Summer Fruit Platter with Crushed Cantucci (page 145)	105
	250 ml/8 fl oz/1 cup skimmed milk for tea and coffee	70
Total		1,190

SUNDAY

		Calories
Breakfast	Banana and Cinnamon Muffin (page 20)	165
Light meal	Ciabatta Pizza with Basil and Sun-dried Tomatoes (page 47)	315
Main meal	Honey-roast Pork Fillet with Orange and Ginger Sauce (page 72)	270
	Celery and Chicory Braise (page 116)	40
Dessert	Poached Pears with Fudgy Chocolate Sauce (page 138)	195
Snack	Feta Cheese Scone (page 144)	90
	250 ml/8 fl oz/1 cup skimmed milk for tea and coffee	70
Total		1,145

NOTES ON THE RECIPES

- All spoon measures are level: 1 tsp = 5ml; 1 tbsp = 15ml.

- Ingredients are given in metric, imperial and American measures. Use only one set per recipe, do not interchange.

- Eggs are medium unless otherwise stated.

- Always wash, peel, core and seed, if necessary, fresh fruit and vegetables before use. Ensure that all produce is as fresh as possible.

- Always use fresh herbs unless dried are specifically called for. If it is necessary to use dried herbs, use half the quantity stated. There is no substitute for fresh parsley and coriander (cilantro).

- All cooking times are approximate and are intended as a guide only.

- Always preheat the oven unless you are using a fan-assisted one and cook on the centre shelf, unless otherwise stated.

- To help you when planning your meals, each recipe shows the percentage of protein, fat, carbohydrate and calorie content in one portion. For those who prefer to use the standard international unit (the joule) to measure energy, one joule is equal to 4.2 calories.

- The recipes and advice given in this book are intended as a guide for those wishing to lose weight in a sensible, realistic way and to maintain a healthy, balanced food intake. If you are worried about any aspect of your health, consult your doctor before embarking on any weight-reducing diet.

HEALTHY BREAKFASTS

Whether you're up at the crack of dawn, or you are a late riser who prefers a more leisurely 'brunch', breakfast is probably the most important meal of the day. It's an essential source of energy for the morning ahead and hopefully will stop you snacking until lunchtime.
You'll find recipes here to suit all tastes, from a fruit compôte, prepared the night before, to a filling platter of rosti with tomatoes and bacon. Try keeping a supply of Blueberry Breakfast Buns (page 19) or Banana and Cinnamon Muffins (page 20) in the freezer to be warmed quickly in the microwave or oven in the morning.
If you prefer, you can simply start the day with a couple of slices of toast with a scraping of low-fat spread, or cereal with skimmed milk. Add a piece of fresh fruit or a small glass of fruit juice, plus a cup of tea or coffee.

Fresh Apple and Hazelnut Muesli

SERVES 1		130 CALORIES PER SERVING
58% CARBOHYDRATE	12% PROTEIN	30% FAT

30 ml/2 tbsp rolled oats

100 ml/3½ fl oz/scant ½ cup skimmed milk

30 ml/2 tbsp condensed milk

1 large eating (dessert) apple

Juice of ½ lemon

15 ml/1 tbsp chopped toasted hazelnuts (filberts)

1 Put the oats in a small bowl and pour over the milk. Cover with clingfilm (plastic wrap) and leave to soak overnight in the fridge.

2 The following day, stir the condensed milk into the soaked oats. Quarter and core and grate the apple and sprinkle with the lemon juice to stop it going brown, then stir into the oat mixture.

3 Sprinkle the chopped toasted hazelnuts over the top and serve straight away, with extra soft fruit, such as raspberries or chopped fresh dates, if liked.

Blueberry Breakfast Buns

MAKES 12		135 CALORIES PER SERVING
65% CARBOHYDRATE	9% PROTEIN	26% FAT

75 g/3 oz/¾ cup self-raising (self-rising) flour

150 g/5 oz/generous 1 cup fine cornmeal

15 ml/1 tbsp baking powder

1.5 ml/¼ tsp salt

50 g/2 oz/¼ cup caster (superfine) sugar

150 ml/¼ pint/⅔ cup skimmed milk

40 g/1½ oz/3 tbsp butter or polyunsaturated spread

Finely grated rind and juice of 1 large orange

1 large egg, beaten

75 g/3 oz/½ cup dried blueberries

1 Sift the flour, cornmeal, baking powder, salt and sugar into a large mixing bowl. Make a well in the middle.

2 Gently heat the milk and butter or spread until melted. Leave to cool, then stir in the orange rind and juice and the beaten egg.

3 Pour into the dry ingredients, add the blueberries and quickly blend together, taking care not to over-mix. Divide the mixture between the sections of a 12-hole muffin tin (pan), lined with paper muffin cases.

4 Bake in a preheated oven at 200°C/400°F/gas mark 6 for 18–20 minutes, or until golden brown and firm. Serve warm or cold.

Banana and Cinnamon Muffins

MAKES 12	165 CALORIES PER SERVING

62% CARBOHYDRATE	12% PROTEIN	26% FAT

175 g/6 oz/1½ cups plain (all-purpose) flour

50 g/2 oz/½ cup plain wholemeal flour

7.5 ml/1½ tsp baking powder

5 ml/1 tsp bicarbonate of soda (baking soda)

5 ml/1 tsp ground cinnamon

50 g/2 oz/½ cup medium oatmeal

50 g/2 oz/¼ cup light Muscovado sugar

25 g/1 oz/¼ cup pecans, roughly chopped

1 egg, beaten

250 ml/8 fl oz/1 cup low-fat plain yoghurt

120 ml/4 fl oz/½ cup skimmed milk

40 g/1½ oz/scant ¼ cup butter or sunflower spread, melted

1 small ripe banana

Greek yoghurt, to serve (optional)

1 Sift the flours, baking powder, bicarbonate of soda and cinnamon into a large mixing bowl, adding the bran left in the sieve (strainer). Stir in the oatmeal, sugar and pecans.

2 Mix together the egg, yoghurt, milk and butter or spread. Peel and mash the banana until smooth, then mix into the egg mixture. Add to the dry ingredients and stir until just blended, taking care not over-mix.

3 Divide the mixture equally between the sections of a 12-hole muffin or deep bun tray lined with paper muffin cases. Bake in a preheated oven at 200°C/400°F/gas mark 6 for about 20 minutes or until well risen and firm.

4 Leave the muffins to cool in the tray for 5 minutes, then transfer to a wire rack. Serve warm or cold with a little Greek yoghurt, if liked.

Fruity Wheatgerm Shake

When you're short of time or simply don't fancy a big breakfast, this nutritious shake makes a great start to the day.

SERVES 1		230 CALORIES PER SERVING
78% CARBOHYDRATE	18% PROTEIN	4% FAT

1 small ripe banana

250 ml/8 fl oz/1 cup chilled skimmed milk

Juice of 1 orange

10 ml/2 tsp clear honey

5 ml/1 tsp wheatgerm

1 Peel the banana and roughly chop. Put in a blender or food processor with all the other ingredients.

2 Whizz the mixture for about 20 seconds or until smooth and frothy. Pour into a tall glass and serve straight away.

Spiced Fruit Compôte with Toasted Nut Topping

SERVES 4		265 CALORIES PER SERVING
69% CARBOHYDRATE	24% FAT	7% PROTEIN

100 g/4 oz/⅔ cup dried apricots

100 g/4 oz/⅔ cup dried apple rings

100 g/4 oz/⅔ cup stoned (pitted) dried prunes

100 g/4 oz/⅔ cup dried figs

1 cinnamon stick

2 whole cloves

1 strip of orange peel

600 ml/1 pt/2½ cups water

For the Toasted Nut Topping:

5 ml/1 tsp water

15 ml/1 tbsp soft light brown sugar

40 g/1½ oz/⅓ cup skinned hazelnuts (filberts), roughly chopped

1 Put all the ingredients for the compôte in a large pan. Slowly bring to the boil and simmer gently for 3 minutes. Remove from the heat, cover with a lid and leave for at least 2 hours.

2 Remove the cinnamon, cloves and orange peel and transfer the compôte to a bowl. Cover and keep in the fridge until ready to serve.

3 For the nut topping, gently heat the water and sugar until the sugar dissolves. Add the hazelnuts and cook for 2 minutes, stirring all the time, until golden brown. Remove from the heat.

4 Remove the compôte from the fridge 30 minutes before serving. Spoon into individual bowls and sprinkle each with a little of the nut topping just before serving.

Creamed Porridge with Peaches

Porridge is rich in vitamins and minerals. It also contains soluble fibre which helps lower blood cholesterol levels.

SERVES 2		280 CALORIES PER SERVING
77% CARBOHYDRATE	16% PROTEIN	7% FAT

100 g/4 oz dried peaches

100 ml/3½ fl oz/scant ½ cup water

30 ml/2 tbsp clear honey

1 vanilla pod

25 g/1 oz/¼ cup porridge oats

450 ml/¾ pt/2 cups skimmed milk

60 ml/4 tbsp no-fat Greek yoghurt

1 Chop the peaches and put in a small pan with the water, honey and vanilla pod. Slowly bring to the boil, then remove from the heat, cover and leave to soak for at least 2 hours or overnight if possible. Remove the vanilla pod.

2 Put the porridge oats in a heavy-based pan. Add the milk and bring to the boil. Simmer for 3 minutes, stirring frequently.

3 Divide the porridge between two bowls and serve each topped with the vanilla-scented peaches and 30 ml/ 2 tbsp Greek yoghurt. Serve straight away.

Tip: Leave the vanilla pod to dry on kitchen paper (paper towels) as it may be used several times.

Rosti with Baked Tomatoes and Crisp Bacon Curls

SERVES 2	200 CALORIES PER SERVING

63% CARBOHYDRATE	18% PROTEIN	19% FAT

350 g/12 oz waxy potatoes, peeled

5 ml/1 tsp sunflower oil

1 small onion, peeled and chopped

30 ml/2 tbsp chopped fresh flatleaf parsley

Salt and freshly ground black pepper

3 tomatoes

2 rashers (slices) of extra-lean back bacon, trimmed

1 Cook the potatoes in boiling salted water for 5 minutes. Drain, cool and coarsely grate.

2 Heat the oil in a non-stick frying pan (skillet) and gently cook the onion for 5 minutes, or until softened and beginning to brown. Mix with the grated potato and chopped parsley and season with salt and pepper.

3 Spoon the mixture into six rounds on a non-stick baking (cookie) tray, flattening slightly with the back of the spoon. Cook in a preheated oven at 200°C/400°F/gas mark 6 for 5 minutes.

4 Cut the tomatoes in half horizontally and season with salt and pepper. Stretch out each rasher of bacon with the back of a knife, then cut into three pieces. Thread concertina-style on to metal skewers.

5 Add the bacon and tomatoes to the baking tray and cook for a further 12–15 minutes, or until the rosti are golden brown and crisp on top and the tomatoes and bacon curls are cooked. Serve the rosti topped with bacon curls and accompanied by the tomatoes.

Smoked Bacon and Avocado Kedgeree

SERVES 2		295 CALORIES PER SERVING
54% CARBOHYDRATE	16% PROTEIN	30% FAT

100 g/4 oz/½ cup long-grain rice

300 ml/½ pt/1¼ cups boiling vegetable stock

1 rasher (slice) of lean smoked back bacon, trimmed and chopped

½ small ripe avocado

15 ml/1 tbsp lemon juice

1 hard-boiled (hard-cooked) egg

30 ml/2 tbsp chopped fresh flatleaf parsley

Salt and freshly ground black pepper

1 Rinse the rice under cold running water and put in a pan. Pour over the boiling stock and bring back to the boil. Stir once, then cover and simmer gently for 15 minutes, until the rice is tender and the stock absorbed.

2 Meanwhile, cook the bacon in a non-stick frying pan (skillet) without adding fat for 3–4 minutes or until crisp. Halve, stone (pit) and chop the avocado and sprinkle with lemon juice, to prevent browning. Shell and chop the egg.

3 As soon as the rice is cooked, stir in the bacon, avocado, egg and parsley. Season to taste with salt and pepper and serve straight away, accompanied by hot unbuttered toast, if liked.

Kidney, Bacon and Mushroom Kebabs

SERVES 2	290 CALORIES PER SERVING	
45% CARBOHYDRATE	30% PROTEIN	25% FAT

2 lambs' kidneys

5 ml/1 tsp plain (all-purpose) flour

A pinch of salt

A little cayenne

4 thin rashers (slices) of lean streaky bacon

8 button mushrooms

5 ml/2 tsp olive oil

5 ml/1 tsp made English mustard

10 ml/2 tsp Worcestershire sauce

5 ml/1 tsp anchovy essence (extract), if liked

5 ml/1 tsp red wine vinegar

5 ml/1 tsp tomato purée (paste)

4 thick slices of wholemeal or granary toast, to serve

1 Skin and halve the kidneys, then snip out the cores with kitchen scissors. Cut each kidney half into two. Lightly dust in the flour, salt and cayenne.

2 Cut each bacon rasher in half and roll up tightly. Thread a bacon roll, then a mushroom and a kidney half on to a skewer, followed by a second bacon roll and another mushroom. Repeat to make another three kebabs.

3 Mix together the olive oil, mustard, Worcestershire sauce, anchovy essence, if using, vinegar and tomato purée. Thickly brush over the kebabs.

4 Put the kebabs on the rack in a grill (broiler) pan. Cook under a preheated medium grill for 4 minutes until beginning to brown, then turn over and cook for another 3 minutes, until tender and browned. Serve the kebabs with hot toast.

Egg, Smoked Salmon and Chive Cocottes

This luxurious recipe for baked eggs is perfect for a celebration breakfast.

SERVES 2		305 CALORIES PER SERVING
44% CARBOHYDRATE	26% PROTEIN	30% FAT

50 g/2 oz smoked salmon

2 eggs

15 ml/1 tbsp snipped fresh chives

15 ml/1 tbsp half-fat crème fraîche

Salt and freshly ground black pepper

4 slices of wholemeal toast, to serve

1 Use the smoked salmon to line the insides of two cocotte dishes or ramekins (custard cups), cutting the salmon to fit.

2 Crack an egg into each dish. Stir the chives into the crème fraîche and season with salt and pepper. Spoon on top of the eggs.

3 Cover the dishes with foil and place on a baking (cookie) sheet. Cook in a preheated oven at 180°C/ 350°F/gas mark 4 for 12–16 minutes, depending how well you like your eggs cooked. Serve hot with fingers of toast.

Fast and Filling

Breakfast is important so don't skip it! To make sure you don't, here are seven simple breakfast ideas, all containing around 150 calories:

- ½ pink grapefruit, plus 1 wholemeal cereal biscuit such as Shredded Wheat or Weetabix, plus 150 ml/¼ pt/⅔ cup skimmed milk.

- 1 small croissant served with 10 ml/2 tsp honey.

- 1 slice of wholemeal or multi-grain bread with a scraping of low-fat spread and 10 ml/2 tsp no-added-sugar jam (conserve) or marmalade, plus 150 ml/¼ pt/⅔ cup unsweetened fruit juice.

- 1 boiled egg with 1 slice of wholemeal toast.

- 25 g/1 oz cornflakes, wheat flakes or rice cereal with 150 ml/¼ pt/⅔ cup skimmed milk.

- 150 ml/¼ pt/⅔ cup low-fat plain or fruit yoghurt with one of the following: 1 apple, pear, peach, orange, or 75 g/3 oz grapes.

- 1 waffle with 15 ml/1 tbsp no-added-sugar jam.

LIGHT LUNCHES AND SIMPLE SUPPERS

Diets are usually planned around the main meal of the day, whether you eat it at midday or in the evening. It's lunch or supper that can be a dieter's downfall. When you're hungry and in a hurry, it's easy to nibble on a few biscuits to fill the gap.

The meals in this chapter solve this problem. Some, such as Saffron and Coriander Steamed Mussels (page 37) can be made in minutes. Others, like Roasted Red Pepper Soup with Garlic Croûtons (page 30) can be made the day before.

If you're working, meals such as Smoked Trout Mousse (page 40) and Mozzarella and Tomato Pan Bagna (page 45) make great packed lunches. If, however, you rely on a snack-bar or canteen, choose low-calorie options such as baked potatoes – don't add butter – with a baked bean or cottage cheese filling. Many shops sell pre-packed calorie-counted sandwiches. If not, chicken or tuna with salad are ideal choices, as long as they're not smothered with mayonnaise.

Roasted Red Pepper Soup with Garlic Croûtons

SERVES 2		230 CALORIES PER SERVING
55% CARBOHYDRATE	15% PROTEIN	30% FAT

2 red (bell) peppers, quartered

1 red chilli, seeded

225 g/8 oz tomatoes, halved

2 garlic cloves, unpeeled

10 ml/2 tsp olive oil

450 ml/¾ pt/2 cups vegetable stock

Salt and freshly ground black pepper

For the Garlic Croûtons:

15 g/½ oz/1 tbsp butter or polyunsaturated margarine

2 garlic cloves, peeled and crushed

4 thick slices of day-old white or wholemeal bread

30 ml/2 tbsp half-fat crème fraîche, to serve

1 Put the peppers, chilli, tomatoes and garlic skin-side up in a single layer in a roasting tin (pan). Drizzle or brush with the olive oil and roast in a preheated oven at 200°C/400°F/gas mark 6 for 45 minutes or until the skins are blistered.

2 Put the peppers and chilli in a polythene bag and leave until cool enough to handle, then peel off the skins. Remove the tomato skins and squeeze the pulp from the garlic.

3 Put the pepper, chilli, tomato and garlic flesh into a food processor with half the stock and blend to a smooth purée. Pour into a saucepan. Stir in the remaining stock and season with salt and pepper. Heat gently until piping hot.

4 Meanwhile, make the Garlic Croûtons. Mix the butter and crushed garlic together, then spread very thinly over one side of each slice of bread.

5 Heat a heavy-based non-stick frying pan (skillet), then add the bread, buttered side down and cook for 2–3 minutes, or until golden brown and crisp. Turn over and cook the other side for 1–2 minutes. Remove from the pan and cut into small cubes.

6 Ladle the soup into warmed bowls and garnish each with a spoonful of half-fat crème fraîche and a few Garlic Croûtons. Serve the remaining croûtons separately.

Chilled Watercress Soup with Cucumber Salsa

SERVES 2		245 CALORIES PER SERVING
50% CARBOHYDRATE	20% PROTEIN	30% FAT

15 ml/1 tbsp sunflower oil

1 leek, thinly sliced

15 ml/1 tbsp plain (all-purpose) flour

300 ml/½ pt/1¼ cups chicken or vegetable stock

150 ml/¼ pt/⅔ cup skimmed milk

Salt and freshly ground black pepper

2 bunches of watercress, about 175 g/6 oz each

For the Cucumber Salsa:

4 spring onions (scallions), thinly sliced

100 g/4 oz cucumber, peeled, seeded and diced

15 ml/1 tbsp lemon juice

5 ml/1 tsp caster sugar

*2 chunks of French bread,
about 50 g/2 oz each, to serve*

1 Heat the oil in a saucepan, add the leek and gently fry (sauté) for 5 minutes, until softened. Stir in the flour and cook gently for 1 minute, stirring.

2 Remove the pan from the heat and gradually stir in the stock, milk and seasoning. Slowly bring to the boil and continue to cook, stirring until slightly thickened.

3 Trim the watercress, discarding any coarse stalks. Roughly chop and stir into the hot soup. Simmer for a few seconds, then leave to cool. Purée in a blender or food processor. Cover and chill for at least 4 hours.

4 Mix together the spring onions, cucumber, lemon juice and sugar with a little salt and pepper in a small bowl. Cover and chill for 1 hour, then drain off any excess liquid.

5 Ladle the chilled soup into individual bowls. Spoon the Cucumber Salsa on top and serve with French bread.

Carrot and Celeriac Soup with Sesame Sticks

SERVES 2		380 CALORIES PER SERVING
58% CARBOHYDRATE	12% PROTEIN	30% FAT

5 ml/1 tsp sunflower oil

1 small onion, finely chopped

175 g/6 oz carrots, grated

175 g/6 oz celeriac (celery root), grated

200 g/7 oz potatoes, diced

450 ml/¾ pt/2 cups vegetable stock

A thinly pared strip of orange rind

30 ml/2 tbsp fresh orange juice

5 ml/1 tsp soy sauce

Salt and freshly ground black pepper

For the Sesame Sticks:

4 thin slices of white bread

15 g/½ oz/2 tbsp butter or polyunsaturated margarine, softened

15 ml/1 tbsp chopped fresh parsley

10 ml/2 tsp sesame seeds

1 Heat the oil in a non-stick saucepan and gently cook the onion for 5 minutes. Add the grated carrots and celeriac, cover the pan and allow the vegetables to steam for 5 minutes, stirring occasionally.

2 Add the potato, stock and orange rind, then cover and simmer for 20 minutes. Stir in the orange juice and soy sauce. Season with salt and pepper to taste.

3 Meanwhile, make the sesame sticks. Trim the crusts off the bread, then roll out firmly with a rolling pin. Mix the butter or margarine, parsley and sesame seeds together and thinly spread two-thirds of the mixture over the bread.

4 Roll up the bread and secure with wooden cocktail sticks (toothpicks). Dot with remaining mixture. Place on a baking (cookie) tray and bake in a preheated oven at 190°C/375°F/gas mark 5 for 15 minutes or until crisp and golden. Remove the cocktail sticks.

5 Ladle the soup into warmed bowls and serve piping hot with the Sesame Sticks.

Pernod-glazed Prawn and Bacon Kebabs

SERVES 2	340 CALORIES PER SERVING

33% CARBOHYDRATE	36% PROTEIN	25% FAT	6% ALCOHOL

4 rashers (slices) of lean back bacon

12 raw tiger prawns (jumbo shrimp), shelled

1 garlic clove, peeled and crushed

2 spring onions (scallions), finely sliced

15 g/½ oz/1 tbsp butter or polyunsaturated margarine

45 ml/3 tbsp Pernod

15 ml/1 tbsp lime juice

Salt and freshly ground black pepper

Lime wedges, to garnish

2 chunks of crusty bread, about 50 g/2 oz each, to serve

1 Remove the rinds and any fat from the bacon. Cut each rasher in half and roll up. Thread two bacon rolls and three prawns on to each of four metal skewers.

2 Gently cook the garlic and spring onions in the butter or margarine for 4 minutes, until softened. Add the Pernod and simmer for a few seconds.

3 Remove from the heat and stir in the lime juice, salt and pepper. Brush a little over the kebabs, then put under a preheated hot grill (broiler) for 3–4 minutes each side or until cooked.

4 Serve the kebabs with the remaining sauce drizzled over. Garnish with wedges of lime and serve with crusty bread to soak up the sauce.

Saffron and Coriander Steamed Mussels

SERVES 2	300 CALORIES PER SERVING
40% CARBOHYDRATE	41% PROTEIN	13% FAT	6% ALCOHOL

150 ml/¼ pt/⅔ cup dry white wine or cider

1 garlic clove, peeled and crushed

1 small onion, finely chopped

1 large pinch of saffron strands

1 kg/2¼ lbs shell-on mussels, scrubbed and bearded

Freshly ground black pepper

45 ml/3 tbsp chopped fresh coriander (cilantro)

2 chunks of French bread, about 50 g/2 oz each, to serve

1 Pour the wine or cider into a large pan. Add the garlic, onion and saffron and bring to the boil. Cover and gently simmer for 5 minutes until the onion is soft.

2 Meanwhile, check the mussels, discarding any that are broken or do not close when tapped. Add to the pan, cover and steam for 4–5 minutes, shaking the pan occasionally. Discard any mussels that have not opened after cooking.

3 Sprinkle the chopped coriander over the mussels and ladle into warmed bowls, leaving in the pan the last couple of spoonfuls of liquid, which may contain some grit. Serve straight away with French bread.

Seared Squid with Chilli Aioli

SERVES 2		435 CALORIES PER SERVING
50% CARBOHYDRATE	21% PROTEIN	29% FAT

175 g/6 oz prepared fresh squid

30 ml/2 tbsp plain (all-purpose) flour

Salt and freshly ground black pepper

2.5 ml/½ tsp Dijon mustard

5 ml/1 tsp lemon juice

1 red chilli, seeded and finely chopped

1 garlic clove, peeled and crushed

45 ml/3 tbsp reduced-fat (light) mayonnaise

15 ml/1 tbsp chopped fresh coriander (cilantro)

10 ml/2 tsp olive oil

Mixed salad leaves

4 slices of French bread, about 2.5 cm/½ in thick, to serve

1 Cut the squid tubes open and lay out flat on a chopping board with the inside uppermost. Lightly score in a criss-cross pattern with a sharp knife.

2 Season the flour with salt and pepper and use to dust the squid. Cut into 2.5 cm/1 in squares.

3 For the Chilli Aioli, blend together the mustard, lemon juice, chilli and garlic. Stir in the mayonnaise and coriander and season with salt and pepper.

4 Heat the oil in a non-stick frying pan (skillet). Add the squid pieces and fry for 1–2 minutes, until firm and just starting to colour.

5 Serve the squid with mixed salad leaves and the Chilli Aioli. Accompany with slices of French bread, toasted.

Butternut Squash and Sweet Potato Soup

SERVES 4		140 CALORIES PER SERVING
89% CARBOHYDRATE	9.5% PROTEIN	1.5% FAT

1 medium onion, roughly chopped

1 garlic clove, peeled and crushed

1 red chilli, seeded and chopped

900 ml/1½ pts/3¾ cups vegetable stock

1 butternut squash, chopped

225 g/8 oz sweet potato, chopped

Salt and freshly ground black pepper

15 ml/1 tbsp chopped fresh flatleaf parsley or coriander (cilantro), to garnish

1 Put the onion, garlic and chilli in a large pan with 150 ml/¼ pt/⅔ cup of the stock. Cover and simmer for 5 minutes, then uncover and simmer until all the liquid has evaporated and the onion is soft.

2 Add the squash, sweet potato and remaining stock to the pan. Bring to the boil, cover and simmer for 20–25 minutes, or until the vegetables are soft.

3 Allow the soup to cool slightly, then purée in batches in a food processor or blender. Return the soup to a clean pan, season with salt and pepper and reheat until piping hot.

4 Ladle the soup into warmed bowls and sprinkle each with chopped fresh parsley or coriander. Serve straight away.

Smoked Trout Mousse with Melba Toast

SERVES 2		195 CALORIES PER SERVING
41% CARBOHYDRATE	39% PROTEIN	20% FAT

75 g/3 oz smoked trout fillet, skinned

100 g/4 oz/½ cup cottage cheese

10 ml/2 tsp lemon juice

White pepper

5 ml/1 tsp powdered gelatine

45 ml/3 tbsp hot vegetable stock or water

15 ml/1 tbsp chopped fresh dill (dill weed)

Lemon wedges and sprigs of fresh dill, to garnish

For the Melba Toast:

3 slices of soft-grain bread

2.5 ml/½ tsp paprika (optional)

1 Roughly chop the smoked trout and put in a blender or food processor with the cottage cheese, lemon juice and pepper. Blend until smooth.

2 Sprinkle the gelatine over the hot stock or water. Stir until dissolved, then leave until just cool. Add to the trout mixture and blend again. Add the chopped dill and blend for just a few seconds to mix.

3 Spoon the mixture into two 150 ml/¼ pt/⅔ cup ramekins (custard cups). Cover with clingfilm (plastic wrap) and chill in the fridge for 2 hours or until set.

4 Meanwhile, make the Melba Toast. Lightly toast the bread on both sides. Cut off the crusts and split each slice into two. Sprinkle with paprika, if liked. Place, untoasted side up, on a grill (broiler) pan under a hot grill and cook for about 1 minute or until brown and crisp.

5 To serve, dip the ramekins (custard cups) into hot water for a few seconds, then turn out on to individual plates. Garnish each with a lemon wedge and a sprig of dill and serve with Melba Toast.

Grilled Potato Wedges with Gorgonzola and Walnut Dip

SERVES 2		365 CALORIES PER SERVING
53% CARBOHYDRATE	17% PROTEIN	30% FAT

2 baking potatoes, about 275 g/10 oz each

Salt and freshly ground black pepper

For the Gorgonzola and Walnut Dip:

40 g/1½ oz Gorgonzola cheese, crumbled

1 small garlic clove, peeled and crushed

100 ml/3½ fl oz/scant ½ cup low-fat fromage frais

15 g/1½ oz toasted walnuts, chopped

1 Cut the potatoes in half lengthways, then in half lengthways again to make four long wedges. Cook in boiling salted water for 4 minutes, then drain thoroughly.

2 Season the potato wedges with a little salt and pepper. Put on a rack over a grill (broiler) pan.

3 Cook under a preheated medium grill for 15 minutes, turning occasionally, until the potatoes are tender and golden brown.

4 Cream the Gorgonzola with the garlic to a smooth paste, then stir in the fromage frais and walnut pieces. Spoon into a bowl and serve with the potato wedges.

Quails' Eggs with Watercress Yoghurt in Crisp Bread Cups

SERVES 2		275 CALORIES PER SERVING
52% CARBOHYDRATE	18% PROTEIN	30% FAT

6 thin slices of white bread

6 quails' eggs

½ bunch of watercress, about 40 g/1½ oz

60 ml/4 tbsp no-fat Greek yoghurt

10 ml/2 tsp lemon juice

Salt and freshly ground black pepper

1 Using a 7.5 cm/3 in plain or fluted biscuit (cookie) cutter, cut out rounds of bread and use to line six sections in a shallow patty tin (pan).

2 Cover each case (shell) with non-stick baking paper and fill with baking beans. Bake for 5 minutes in a preheated oven at 200°C/400°F/gas mark 6, then remove the paper and beans and cook for a further 5 minutes until golden brown and crisp.

3 Meanwhile, cook the quails' eggs in boiling water for 45 seconds. Remove and cool them under cold running water. Carefully shell the eggs, then cut in half lengthways.

4 Trim the watercress and remove any coarse stalks. Finely chop the rest and mix with the yoghurt, lemon juice, salt and pepper.

5 Arrange two egg halves in each bread cup, cut side uppermost, then spoon over the Watercress Yoghurt. Once filled, serve straight away.

Oriental Chicken Skewers with Sesame Noodles

SERVES 2		430 CALORIES PER PERSON
51% CARBOHYDRATE	25% PROTEIN	24% FAT

225 g/8 oz skinless chicken breast fillets

2.5 cm/1 in piece of fresh root ginger

1 garlic clove

30 ml/2 tbsp dry sherry

30 ml/2 tbsp dark soy sauce

5 ml/1 tsp clear honey

For the Sesame Noodles:

225 g/8 oz egg noodles

15 ml/1 tbsp sesame seeds

5 ml/1 tsp sesame oil

1 Slice the chicken into finger-length strips, about 1 cm/ ½ in wide. Peel and finely grate the ginger and crush the garlic.

2 Mix the ginger, garlic, sherry, soy sauce and honey in a bowl. Add the chicken and turn to coat thoroughly. Cover with clingfilm (plastic wrap) and marinate in the fridge for at least 3 hours or overnight. Meanwhile, soak six wooden satay sticks in water (this helps stop them burning during cooking).

3 Thread the chicken strips on to the satay sticks and arrange on a grill (broiler) pan. Cover the exposed part of the sticks with foil. Cook under a hot grill for 12–15 minutes, turning occasionally and brushing with any remaining marinade.

4 Meanwhile, cook the noodles in boiling salted water according to the packet instructions. Drain thoroughly. Toast the sesame seeds in a non-stick pan over a medium heat for 2–3 minutes, stirring all the time until golden brown.

5 Toss the toasted sesame seeds and oil with the noodles. Pile on to two warmed plates, topping each with two chicken skewers. Serve straight away.

Mozzarella and Tomato Pan Bagna

SERVES 2		450 CALORIES PER SERVING
54% CARBOHYDRATE	25% PROTEIN	21% FAT

1 small French stick

225 g/8 oz plum or beefsteak tomatoes, sliced

Salt and freshly ground black pepper

100 g/4 oz reduced-fat (light) Mozzarella cheese, sliced

1 little gem lettuce, shredded

50 g/2 oz stoned (pitted) black olives

A few torn basil leaves

1 With a sharp serrated knife, cut the French stick in half, then slice lengthways and open out.

2 Sprinkle the tomato slices with salt and pepper.

3 Fill the bread with a layer of tomatoes, followed by slices of Mozzarella and a scattering of shredded lettuce, olives and basil.

4 Wrap tightly in clingfilm (plastic wrap) and chill for at least 30 minutes to allow the flavours to develop.

Garlic Mushrooms and Dill Dip

SERVES 3		235 CALORIES PER SERVING
48% CARBOHYDRATE	22% PROTEIN	30% FAT

75 g/3 oz/1½ cups fresh white breadcrumbs

15 g/½ oz/1 tbsp freshly grated Parmesan

2.5 ml/½ tsp paprika

Salt and freshly ground black pepper

1 egg white

175 g/6 oz button mushrooms

15 g/½ oz/1 tbsp butter or sunflower spread

1 garlic clove, peeled and crushed

For the Dill Dip:

50 g/2 oz/¼ cup low-fat curd cheese

60 ml/4 tbsp no-fat Greek yoghurt

30 ml/2 tbsp chopped fresh dill (dill weed)

1 Mix together the breadcrumbs, Parmesan, paprika, salt and pepper in a bowl. Lightly whisk the egg white with a fork, then dip the mushrooms, one at a time, first into the egg white, then into the breadcrumbs. Place on a non-stick baking (cookie) sheet.

2 Melt the butter or sunflower spread and mix with the crushed garlic. Drizzle a little on top of each mushroom. Bake in a preheated oven at 180°C/350°F/ gas mark 4 for 15–20 minutes or until the mushrooms are tender and the coating lightly browned.

3 Meanwhile, mix together all the ingredients for the Dill Dip. Spoon into a small bowl and garnish with dill. Put on a plate and surround with the hot garlic mushrooms. Serve straight away.

Ciabatta Pizza with Basil and Sun-dried Tomatoes

SERVES 4		315 CALORIES PER SERVING
53% CARBOHYDRATE	17% PROTEIN	30% FAT

1 ciabatta loaf

15 ml/1 tbsp oil from the sun-dried tomatoes

450 g/1 lb ripe plum or beefsteak tomatoes, thinly sliced

2 garlic cloves, peeled and finely chopped

100 g/4 oz yellow cherry tomatoes, halved

50 g/2 oz sun-dried tomatoes in oil, drained and sliced

50 g/2 oz Parmesan cheese

Salt and freshly ground black pepper

A few torn basil leaves

1 Cut the loaf in half horizontally. Brush each cut surface with the oil and lightly toast the cut side under a hot grill (broiler).

2 Arrange the tomato slices over the ciabatta, then the garlic and the cherry and sun-dried tomatoes. Using a potato peeler, shave Parmesan over the top.

3 Put the pizza on a baking (cookie) sheet and cook in a preheated oven at 200°C/400°F/gas mark 6 for 15 minutes. Serve straight away.

Red Bean Burritos

SERVES 2	290 CALORIES PER SERVING

59% CARBOHYDRATE	20% PROTEIN	21% FAT

10 ml/2 tsp olive oil

1 small red onion, finely chopped

1 garlic clove, peeled and crushed

1 red chilli, seeded and finely chopped

200 g/7 oz/1 small can of chopped tomatoes with herbs

200 g/7 oz/1 small can of red kidney beans, drained

5 ml/1 tsp tomato purée (paste)

Salt and freshly ground black pepper

2 ready-made flour tortillas

25 g/1 oz/¼ cup grated Gruyère cheese

*Green salad and 60 ml/4 tbsp thick plain yoghurt,
to serve*

1 Heat the oil in a saucepan and gently fry (sauté) the onion for 5 minutes. Add the garlic and chilli and fry for 5 more minutes, or until the onion is very soft.

2 Stir in the chopped tomatoes and simmer for 15 minutes or until the sauce is thick. Stir in the kidney beans, tomato purée, salt and pepper.

3 Divide the sauce between the tortillas, spreading it almost to the edges. Sprinkle over half of the cheese, then roll up the tortillas. Put seam-side down in a shallow baking dish.

4 Sprinkle the rest of the cheese over the tortillas. Bake in a preheated oven at 200°C/400°F/gas mark 6 for 15 minutes or until the cheese is bubbling. Serve with the green salad and yoghurt.

MEAT AND FISH MAIN MEALS

Meat is an excellent source of protein and provides iron in a form that the body can easily use, as well as B-vitamins and minerals. However, it can also be a source of large quantities of saturated fat in our diet, so this chapter contains recipes for leaner cuts of beef, lamb and pork and also lots of tempting ideas for poultry.

We don't need to eat a great deal of meat; a 100 g/4 oz serving provides more than half of our daily requirements of protein. To satisfy healthy appetites, make a little meat go a long way by adding starchy carbohydrates such as rice, pasta and potatoes.

Fish is a wonderful choice for slimmers. It has the benefits of being not only high in protein like meat, but also much lower in fat. For both fish and meat, the lowest-calorie cooking methods are grilling (broiling), poaching and baking, which bring out their natural flavours.

Chicken with Roasted Fennel and Baked Lemon Rice

SERVES 2		475 CALORIES PER SERVING
36% CARBOHYDRATE	35% PROTEIN	29% FAT

5 ml/1 tsp fennel seeds

15 ml/1 tbsp chopped fresh oregano

1 garlic clove, peeled and crushed

Salt and freshly ground black pepper

2 chicken breasts, 175 g/6 oz each, with wings attached

1 fennel bulb

10 ml/2 tsp olive oil

100 g/4 oz/½ cup long-grain rice

Finely grated rind and juice of ½ lemon

300 ml/½ pt/1¼ cups chicken or vegetable stock

6 black olives, stoned (pitted)

1 Lightly crush the fennel seeds and mix with the oregano, garlic, salt and pepper.

2 Tuck the fennel seed and garlic mixture between the skin and flesh of the chicken breasts, keeping the skin intact. Place on a baking (cookie) tray.

3 Trim the fennel bulb and cut into eight wedges. Brush the oil over the fennel and add to the tray with the chicken. Bake on the top shelf of a preheated oven at 220ºC/425ºF/gas mark 7 for 5 minutes.

4 Meanwhile, put the rice in a 1.2 litre/2 pt/5 cup ovenproof casserole (Dutch oven). Stir in the lemon rind and juice and the stock and season with salt and pepper. Cover and put on the shelf below the chicken.

5 Turn down the oven to 180°C/350°F/gas mark 4 and cook for a further 40–45 minutes or until cooked, turning the fennel once during cooking. Add the olives to the chicken 5 minutes before the end of cooking time.

6 Fluff up the Lemon Rice with a fork and serve topped with the chicken and fennel.

Cream Cheese and Peanut Chicken Bites

SERVES 2		530 CALORIES PER SERVING
50% CARBOHYDRATE	27% PROTEIN	23% FAT

200 g/7 oz chicken breast meat

25 g/1 oz/½ cup fresh white breadcrumbs

15 ml/1 tbsp half-fat cream cheese

15 ml/1 tbsp peanut butter

1 egg

30 ml/2 tbsp chopped fresh flatleaf parsley

Salt and freshly ground black pepper

175 g/6 oz tagliatelle

Green vegetable or side salad, to serve

1 Roughly chop the chicken and put in a food processor with the breadcrumbs, cream cheese, peanut butter, egg, parsley, salt and pepper. Process until fairly chunky.

2 Drop spoonfuls of the mixture on to a lightly greased non-stick baking (cookie) tray – it will make about ten. Bake at 180°C/350°C/gas mark 4 for 15 minutes until golden brown and cooked.

3 Meanwhile, cook the tagliatelle in boiling salted water according to the packet instructions. Drain well. Pile on to two warmed plates with the chicken bites and serve with a green vegetable or a side salad.

Chicken Cacciatora

SERVES 2   465 CALORIES PER SERVING

33% CARBOHYDRATE   35% PROTEIN   25% FAT   7% ALCOHOL

10 ml/2 tsp olive oil

4 chicken thighs, boned

1 garlic clove, peeled and crushed

A sprig of fresh rosemary

A sprig of fresh thyme

100 ml/3½ fl oz/scant ½ cup dry white wine

60 ml/4 tbsp chicken stock

200 g/7 oz/1 small can of chopped tomatoes

25 g/1 oz stoned (pitted) black olives

15 g/½ oz capers, drained

Salt and freshly ground black pepper

Sprigs of fresh rosemary, to garnish

2 ciabatta rolls and green salad, to serve

1   Heat the oil in a heavy non-stick frying pan (skillet) to a moderate heat, then add the chicken thighs. Cook for 3–4 minutes until browned, then turn over, add the garlic and herbs and cook for a further 3–4 minutes.

2   Pour in the wine and simmer for 3 minutes to reduce slightly. Add the stock and tomatoes, cover and gently simmer for 15 minutes.

3   Stir in the olives and capers. Season to taste with salt and pepper. Cook, uncovered, for a further 5 minutes or until the sauce is thick and the chicken tender.

4   Spoon on to plates, garnish with sprigs of fresh rosemary and serve with the warm ciabatta rolls and a green side salad, if liked.

Herby Baked Chicken and Oven Fries

SERVES 2		550 CALORIES PER SERVING
42% CARBOHYDRATE	29% PROTEIN	29% FAT

4 chicken drumsticks, skin removed

15 ml/1 tbsp seasoned flour

50 g/2 oz/1 cup fine fresh white breadcrumbs

15 ml/1 tbsp finely grated Parmesan cheese

2.5 ml/½ tsp paprika

2.5 ml/½ tsp dried mixed herbs

1 egg, beaten

For the Oven Fries:

350 g/12 oz potatoes

600 ml/1 pt/2½ cups boiling vegetable stock

15 ml/1 tbsp sunflower oil

Flatleaf parsley and lemon wedges, to garnish

1 Roll the drumsticks in the flour to coat. Put the breadcrumbs, cheese, paprika and herbs in a shallow bowl and mix together.

2 Dip the floured drumsticks in the beaten egg, then in the breadcrumb mixture to coat. Arrange on a non-stick baking (cookie) tray. Bake on the middle shelf of a preheated oven at 200°C/400°F/gas mark 6 for 30 minutes.

3 Meanwhile, peel the potatoes and cut into thick chips (fries). Add to a pan containing the boiling stock and simmer for 3 minutes or until almost tender. Drain well.

4 Put the chips in a large bowl and drizzle over the oil. Toss until lightly coated. Tip on to a non-stick baking tray.

5 Bake the chips on the top shelf of the oven, above the chicken, for 15 minutes or until crisp and golden, turning once or twice during cooking.

6 Sprinkle the Oven Fries with a little salt and serve on warmed plates with the chicken, garnished with flatleaf parsley and lemon wedges.

Pan-fried Chicken with Thai Spices

SERVES 2		475 CALORIES PER SERVING
33% CARBOHYDRATE	37% PROTEIN	30% FAT

2.5 cm/1 in piece of root ginger, peeled and chopped

3 kaffir lime leaves

150 ml/¼ pt/⅔ cup chicken stock

2 chicken breasts, 75 g/6 oz each, skinned

5 ml/1 tsp groundnut (peanut) oil

60 ml/4 tbsp coconut milk

10 ml/2 tsp Thai fish sauce

1 red chilli, seeded and finely chopped

100 g/4 oz Thai jasmine rice

15 ml/1 tbsp lime juice

30 ml/2 tbsp chopped fresh coriander (cilantro)

1   Put the ginger and kaffir lime leaves in a bowl. Bring the chicken stock to the boil and pour over. Leave to infuse for 20 minutes.

2   Meanwhile, cut each chicken breast into two pieces. Heat the oil in a flameproof casserole (Dutch oven) and brown the chicken pieces for 2–3 minutes each side.

3   Strain the infused chicken stock into the pan. Cover and simmer for 15 minutes. Stir in the coconut milk, fish sauce and chilli. Simmer, uncovered, for 4–5 minutes, until the chicken is cooked and the sauce reduced slightly.

4   Meanwhile, cook the rice in boiling salted water according to the packet instructions. Drain well and spoon on to warmed plates. Stir the lime juice and coriander into the chicken and serve on a bed of rice.

Citrus Chicken Schnitzel

SERVES 2		475 CALORIES PER SERVING
62% CARBOHYDRATE	30% PROTEIN	8% FAT

225 g/8 oz boneless chicken breasts, skinned

Juice of ½ lemon

30 ml/2 tbsp orange juice

30 ml/2 tbsp plain (all-purpose) flour

1.5 ml/¼ tsp dried mixed herbs

2.5 ml/½ tsp celery salt

Freshly ground black pepper

1 egg, beaten

40 g/1½ oz/generous ¼ cup fine dry breadcrumbs

100 g/4 oz/½ cup long-grain and wild rice

Green vegetable, to serve

1 Cut the chicken breasts horizontally into 5 mm/¼ in slices. Place between greaseproof or non-stick baking paper and beat gently with a rolling pin to flatten.

2 Put the chicken in a shallow dish and sprinkle with the lemon and orange juices. Leave to marinate for 20 minutes.

3 Combine the flour, herbs, celery salt and pepper on a plate. Dip the chicken in the flour mixture, then in the beaten egg and finally in the breadcrumbs to coat.

4 Put the chicken on a non-stick baking (cookie) tray and bake in a preheated oven at 200°C/400°F/gas mark 6 for 10–12 minutes until browned and cooked through.

5 Cook the rice in boiling salted water for 10 minutes, or according to the packet instructions. Drain well. Serve the chicken with the rice and a green vegetable.

Creamy Chicken Korma

SERVES 2		540 CALORIES PER SERVING
42% CARBOHYDRATE	33% PROTEIN	25% FAT

15 g/½ oz/2 tbsp desiccated (shredded) coconut

15 ml/1 tbsp sunflower oil

1 onion, finely chopped

2 garlic cloves, peeled and crushed

2 whole cloves

2.5 cm/1 in piece of root ginger, peeled and grated

5 ml/1 tsp ground coriander (cilantro)

2.5 ml/½ tsp ground cumin

1.5 ml/¼ tsp ground turmeric

2 boneless chicken breasts, all skin removed

15 ml/1 tbsp lemon juice

300 ml/½ pt/1¼ cups thick plain yoghurt

2.5 ml/½ tsp cornflour (cornstarch)

Salt and freshly ground black pepper

100 g/4 oz/½ cup basmati rice

30 ml/2 tbsp chopped fresh coriander

Sprigs of fresh coriander, to serve

1 Put the coconut in a small bowl and pour over 75 ml/ 5 tbsp boiling water. Leave to soak for at least 10 minutes. Heat the oil in a large frying pan (skillet) and gently fry (sauté) the onion for 10 minutes, until very soft.

2 Add the garlic, cloves, ginger, ground coriander, cumin and turmeric to the pan and cook for 2 minutes, stirring all the time.

3 Cut the chicken into 2.5 cm/1 in cubes. Add to the pan with the lemon juice. Turn down the heat and gradually stir in the yoghurt, a spoonful at a time.

4 Drain the coconut, reserving the liquid. Blend the cornflour with the liquid and stir into the chicken mixture. Season with salt and pepper.

5 Half-cover the pan with a lid and cook very gently for 30 minutes, or until the chicken is cooked through. Remove the cloves. Meanwhile, cook the rice in boiling salted water for 10–12 minutes, until tender. Drain thoroughly.

6 Spoon the rice on to two warmed plates. Stir the fresh chopped coriander into the chicken korma and spoon over the rice. Serve garnished with sprigs of fresh coriander.

Chicken and Wild Mushroom Lasagne

SERVES 2		510 CALORIES PER SERVING
35% CARBOHYDRATE	35% PROTEIN	30% FAT

15 g/½ oz/1 tbsp butter or polyunsaturated margarine

25 g/1 oz/¼ cup plain (all-purpose) flour

300 ml/½ pt/1¼ cups skimmed milk

1 bay leaf

100 g/4 oz mixed wild mushrooms

10 ml/2 tsp olive oil

175 g/6 oz/1½ cups chopped cooked chicken

1.5 ml/¼ tsp grated nutmeg

Salt and freshly ground black pepper

200 g/7 oz/1 small can of plum tomatoes, drained and chopped

2.5 ml/½ tsp dried oregano or mixed herbs

4 sheets of no-need-to-precook lasagne

1 egg, beaten

150 ml/¼ pt/⅔ cup no-fat Greek yoghurt

15g ml/1 tbsp grated Parmesan or Pecorino Romano cheese

Green salad, to serve

1 For the sauce, put the butter or margarine, flour, milk and bay leaf in a pan. Slowly bring to the boil, stirring until thickened. Simmer for 4–5 minutes. Remove the bay leaf.

2 Slice the mushrooms and cook in the oil in a non-stick frying pan (skillet) for 3 minutes. Stir into the sauce with the chicken and nutmeg. Season to taste with salt and pepper. Mix the chopped tomatoes and dried herbs together.

3 Spoon the tomato mixture into the base of a 900 ml/ 1½ pt/3¾ cup rectangular ovenproof dish. Top with two sheets of lasagne. Spoon in the chicken and mushroom sauce. Top with the remaining sheets of lasagne.

4 Mix together the egg, yoghurt and Parmesan or Pecorino Romano cheese. Season with salt and pepper and spread over the top. Bake at 180°C/350°F/gas mark 5 for 40–45 minutes or until the lasagne is tender and the top is golden brown and set. Serve hot with a green salad.

Teriyaki Turkey with Oriental Noodles

SERVES 2		510 CALORIES PER SERVING
56% CARBOHYDRATE	14% PROTEIN	30% FAT

45 ml/3 tbsp Japanese soy sauce

30 ml/2 tbsp sake or dry sherry

10 ml/2 tsp caster (superfine) sugar

225 g/8 oz turkey breast meat

150 g/5 oz medium egg noodles

10 ml/2 tsp sesame oil

1 garlic clove, peeled and crushed

5 ml/1 tsp chopped fresh root ginger

1 medium carrot, cut into fine strips

1 courgette (zucchini), cut into fine strips

15 ml/1 tbsp toasted sesame seeds

1 Put the soy sauce, sake or sherry and sugar in a small saucepan and heat gently until the sugar has dissolved. Allow to cool.

2 Cut the turkey into strips and put in a shallow bowl with the soy mixture. Toss to coat, cover and leave to marinate in the fridge for 2 hours. Meanwhile, soak four bamboo skewers in cold water.

3 Thread the marinated turkey on to the skewers, reserving the marinade.

4 Cook the egg noodles in a large pan of boiling salted water according to the packet instructions. Drain well.

5 Cook the turkey skewers under a preheated hot grill (broiler) for 6–7 minutes, turning and basting with the marinade, until the turkey is cooked through.

6 Heat the sesame oil in a large non-stick frying pan (skillet) or wok and cook the garlic and ginger for a few seconds. Add the carrot and courgette and cook for 3 minutes. Add any remaining marinade to the pan and simmer for a few seconds.

7 Add the noodles to the pan, gently toss and heat through. Pile on to warmed plates and top each with two turkey skewers. Sprinkle with sesame seeds and serve straight away.

Duck Satay with Aromatic Rice

SERVES 2		375 CALORIES PER SERVING
45% CARBOHYDRATE	27% PROTEIN	28% FAT

175 g/6 oz boneless duck breast, skinned

1.5 ml/¼ tsp ground ginger

15 ml/1 tbsp dry sherry

15 ml/1 tbsp soy sauce

Finely grated rind and juice of 1 orange

Freshly ground black pepper

900 ml/1½ pts/3¾ cups vegetable or chicken stock

1.5 ml/¼ tsp salt

1 star anise

½ stick of cinnamon

75 g/3 oz/⅓ cup brown rice

40 g/1½ oz/⅓ cup unsalted cashew nuts

30 ml/2 tbsp chopped fresh coriander (cilantro)

1 Cut the duck into bite-sized cubes. Mix the ginger, sherry, soy sauce, orange rind and juice in a bowl. Stir in the duck, cover and marinate in the fridge for 2 hours. Put four wooden skewers into cold water to soak.

2 Bring the stock and salt to the boil in a large pan. Add the star anise, cinnamon stick and rice. Cover and cook for about 25 minutes or until the rice is tender. Drain well.

3 Meanwhile, thread the duck on to the skewers. Put them in a roasting tin (pan), pour in the remaining marinade and cook in a preheated oven at 200°C/400°F/gas mark 6 for 10 minutes or until the duck is cooked and tender.

4 Put the cashew nuts in a food processor or blender with the cooking juices from the duck and blend until smooth. Put in a small serving bowl.

5 Remove the spices from the rice and stir in the chopped coriander. Spoon on to warmed plates, top with the duck and serve with the cashew nut satay sauce.

Lamb Cutlets with Hot Apricot Tabbouleh

SERVES 2		305 CALORIES PER SERVING
50% CARBOHYDRATE	25% PROTEIN	25% FAT

4 lean lamb cutlets, about 100 g/4 oz each

1 garlic clove, peeled and halved

10 ml/2 tsp clear honey

10 ml/2 tsp chopped mixed fresh herbs, eg thyme, rosemary and oregano

Salt and freshly ground black pepper

For the Hot Apricot Tabbouleh:

600 ml/1 pt/2½ cups vegetable stock

75 g/3 oz/½ cup bulgar (cracked) wheat

175 g/6 oz fresh apricots

4 spring onions (scallions)

10 ml/2 tsp olive oil

10 ml/2 tsp lemon juice

1 Trim all the fat off the lamb cutlets and rub them with the cut side of the garlic clove. Brush both sides of the cutlets with the honey and sprinkle with the herbs and a little salt and pepper. Put on a grill (broiler) pan.

2 Bring the vegetable stock to the boil in a saucepan. Add the bulgar wheat and turn off the heat. Cover and leave to soak for 15 minutes.

3 Half and dice the fresh apricots. Trim and slice the spring onions diagonally. Heat the oil in a frying pan (skillet) and gently cook the spring onions for 3–4 minutes. Add the apricots and cook for about 30 seconds.

4 Bring the bulgar wheat back to the boil, then drain well. Stir in the spring onions, apricots and lemon juice. Season to taste with salt and pepper.

5 Meanwhile, cook the lamb cutlets under a preheated hot grill for 8–10 minutes, until browned and tender. Spoon the bulgar wheat on to warmed plates and top with the cutlets.

Spiced Lamb Skewers with Golden Rice and Minted Yoghurt

SERVES 2		450 CALORIES PER SERVING
37% CARBOHYDRATE	31% PROTEIN	32% FAT

225 g/8 oz lean minced (ground) lamb

1 garlic clove, crushed

2.5 cm/1 in piece of fresh root ginger, peeled and grated

5 ml/1 tsp medium curry paste

1 egg yolk

Salt and freshly ground black pepper

100 g/4 oz/½ cup long-grain rice

2.5 ml/½ tsp ground turmeric

30 ml/2 tbsp chopped fresh mint

150 ml/¼ pt/⅔ cup no-fat Greek yoghurt

Sprigs of fresh mint, to garnish

1 Mix together the minced lamb with the garlic, ginger, curry paste, egg yolk, salt and pepper. Shape the mixture into 12 balls and thread on to two metal skewers.

2 Preheat the grill (broiler) to high and cook the lamb skewers for 10–15 minutes, turning until browned all over and cooked through.

3 Meanwhile, cook the rice and turmeric in boiling salted water for 10 minutes, or until tender. Drain well. Stir the chopped mint into the yoghurt. Spoon into a serving bowl.

4 Spoon the rice on to warmed individual plates and top each with a lamb skewer. Serve with the minted yoghurt garnished with sprigs of fresh mint.

Gammon with Pineapple Relish

SERVES 2   530 CALORIES PER SERVING

40% CARBOHYDRATE   43% PROTEIN   17% FAT

2 gammon steaks, about 175 g/6 oz each

Freshly ground black pepper

200 g/7 oz/1 small can of pineapple chunks in natural juice, drained and roughly chopped

10 ml/2 tsp soft light brown sugar

10 ml/2 tsp white wine vinegar

30 ml/2 tbsp finely chopped preserved ginger

15 ml/1 tbsp syrup from the ginger

15 ml/1 tbsp chopped fresh flatleaf parsley

100 g/4 oz/½ cup long-grain and wild rice

Salt

Broccoli, to serve

1 Put the gammon steaks on a grill (broiler) pan and season with a little black pepper.

2 Put the pineapple in a pan with the sugar, vinegar, ginger and syrup. Bring to the boil and simmer, uncovered, for 15 minutes or until all the liquid has evaporated. Stir in the parsley and season to taste with pepper.

3 Cook the rice in boiling salted water according to the packet instructions. Drain well. Meanwhile, cook the gammon steaks under a preheated hot grill (broiler) for 3–4 minutes each side until cooked through.

4 Transfer the gammon steaks to warmed plates and serve with the rice and broccoli. Accompany with the Pineapple Relish, either warm or cold.

Pork and Orchard Fruit in Cider Sauce with Mustard Mash

SERVES 2		430 CALORIES PER SERVING
52% CARBOHYDRATE	23% PROTEIN	20% FAT 5% ALCOHOL

100 g/4 oz/⅔ cup dried fruit salad

150 ml/¼ pt/⅔ cup medium cider

15 ml/1 tbsp sunflower oil

175 g/6 oz lean pork steak, cut into strips

1 small onion, sliced

1.5 ml/¼ tsp ground allspice

10 ml/2 tsp cornflour (cornstarch)

200 ml/7 fl oz/scant 1 cup vegetable stock

Salt and freshly ground black pepper

15 ml/1 tbsp chopped fresh parsley

For the Mustard Mash:

225 g/8 oz potatoes, peeled

45 ml/3 tbsp skimmed milk

15 ml/1 tbsp wholegrain mustard

1 Put the dried fruit in a small saucepan with the cider and slowly bring to the boil. Remove from the heat, cover with a lid and leave to soak for 1 hour.

2 Heat 10 ml/2 tsp oil in a non-stick frying pan (skillet) and cook the pork for 2–3 minutes, stirring, until browned all over. Transfer to a flameproof casserole (Dutch oven).

3 Heat the remaining 5 ml/1 tsp oil and gently cook the onion for 10 minutes, until beginning to colour. Stir in the allspice and cook for a few seconds, then add to the casserole.

4 Blend the cornflour with 30 ml/2 tbsp soaking liquid from the fruit. Stir into the stock. Add the stock to the casserole with the fruit and soaking liquid, salt and pepper.

5 Bring to the boil, stirring until thickened. Cover and cook in a preheated oven at 180°C/350°F/gas mark 4 for 45 minutes, or until the pork is tender. Stir in the chopped parsley.

6 Meanwhile, make the Mustard Mash. Cut the potatoes into large chunks and cook in boiling salted water for 15 minutes, or until tender. Drain well and mash with the milk and mustard and season with black pepper. Serve with the pork.

Honey-roast Pork Fillet with Orange and Ginger Sauce

SERVES 2		270 CALORIES PER SERVING
54% CARBOHYDRATE	33% PROTEIN	13% FAT

1.5 ml/¼ tsp whole tropical peppercorns

15 ml/1 tbsp thick honey

5 ml/1 tsp soy sauce

5 ml/1 tsp chopped fresh rosemary

175 g/6 oz pork tenderloin

For the Orange and Ginger Sauce:

2 oranges

2 thin slices of fresh root ginger

5 ml/1 tsp cornflour (cornstarch)

A pinch of salt

200 g/8 oz new potatoes, to serve

1 Lightly crush the peppercorns. Mix the honey, soy sauce and rosemary in a small bowl and brush all over the pork, then sprinkle with the peppercorns.

2 Put the pork in a non-stick roasting tin (pan) and cook in a preheated oven at 180°C/350°F/gas mark 4 for 25–30 minutes or until cooked through. Cover and 'rest' in a warm place for 10 minutes.

3 Meanwhile, make the sauce; thinly pare a strip of rind from the orange and cut into julienne strips. Squeeze the juice from the same orange and put into a small saucepan, with the ginger. Cover and simmer for 5 minutes.

4 Peel the remaining orange, removing all the white pith. Remove the segments by cutting between the membranes, holding the fruit over a bowl to catch the juices.

5 Blend the cornflour with 15 ml/1 tbsp cold water. Add to the pan and simmer for 1 minute, until thickened. Stir in the orange segments and juice. Season with salt and gently heat through.

6 Cut the pork into slices and arrange on warmed plates. Spoon the sauce over and serve with boiled new potatoes and green beans.

Pesto Pork with Tomato Rice

SERVES 2		395 CALORIES PER SERVING
42% CARBOHYDRATE	28% PROTEIN	30% FAT

For the Tomato Rice:

10 ml/2 tsp olive oil

½ small red onion, finely chopped

15 ml/1 tbsp sun-dried tomato purée (paste)

75 g/3 oz/scant ½ cup long-grain rice

250 ml/8 fl oz/1 cup vegetable or chicken stock

2.5 ml/½ tsp salt and freshly ground black pepper

For the Pesto Pork:

150 g/5 oz pork fillet

25 g/1 oz/2 tbsp half-fat cream cheese

30 ml/2 tbsp pesto sauce

1 egg, beaten

15 ml/1 tbsp finely grated Parmesan cheese

1 Heat the oil in a non-stick frying pan (skillet) and gently cook the onion for 5 minutes, until beginning to soften. Stir in the sun-dried tomato purée and rice and cook for 1 minute, stirring.

2 Remove from the heat and stir in the stock. Season with salt and pepper and transfer to a 1.2 litre/2 pt/ 5 cup flameproof casserole (Dutch oven).

3 Cover with a lid or foil and cook on the middle shelf in a preheated oven at 180°C/350°F/gas mark 4 for 40 minutes, or until the rice is tender and the stock absorbed.

4 Meanwhile, slit the pork fillet almost in half lengthways and open up. Mix the cream cheese and pesto and spread down the middle, then fold the pork over to enclose the filling. Tie at intervals with fine string.

5 Brush the outside with beaten egg and roll in Parmesan to coat. Cook in a roasting tin (pan) on the top shelf of the oven, for 25–30 minutes, or until cooked through. Cover, 'rest' for 5 minutes, then slice. Serve with the Tomato Rice.

Braised Steak in Burgundy with Filo Topping

SERVES 2   475 CALORIES PER SERVING

45% CARBOHYDRATE   29% PROTEIN   19% FAT   7% ALCOHOL

1 small red onion, thinly sliced

100 ml/3½ fl oz/scant ½ cup beef stock

225 g/8 oz lean chuck steak

15 ml/1 tbsp plain (all-purpose) flour

100 ml/3½ fl oz/scant ½ cup burgundy or other red wine

100 g/4 oz baby button mushrooms

50 g/2 oz/3 sheets of filo pastry (paste)

10 ml/2 tsp sunflower oil

*2 baked potatoes, about 100 g/4 oz each,
and broccoli, to serve*

1 Put the onion in a non-stick frying pan (skillet) with half the stock. Cover with a lid and simmer for 5 minutes, then uncover and simmer until all the stock has evaporated. Remove from the pan and set aside.

2 Trim any visible fat from the beef and cut into 2.5cm/ 1 in cubes. Dry-fry the meat in a non-stick frying pan until lightly browned. Sprinkle over the flour and stir in. Add the onion and stir in the remaining stock and the red wine.

3 Slowly bring to the boil, stirring all the time. Cover and simmer very gently for 1 hour. Stir in the mushrooms and cook for a further 20–25 minutes, or until the meat is tender. Spoon into a 750 ml/1¼ pt/3 cup pie dish.

4   Brush a sheet of the filo with a little of the oil. Crumple it loosely and arrange, oiled side up, on top of the meat. Repeat with the remaining pastry and oil.

5   Bake in a preheated oven at 180°C/350°F/gas mark 4 for 25–30 minutes, or until the pastry is lightly browned and crisp. Serve with baked potatoes and broccoli.

Beef with Red Peppers in Paprika Sauce

SERVES 2		460 CALORIES PER SERVING
42% CARBOHYDRATE	28% PROTEIN	30% FAT

100 g/4 oz/½ cup long-grain and wild rice

225 g/8 oz rump steak

10 ml/2 tsp olive oil

1 bunch of spring onions (scallions), trimmed and sliced

1 small red (bell) pepper, sliced

5 ml/1 tsp paprika

Salt and freshly ground black pepper

60 ml/4 tbsp half-fat crème fraîche

30 ml/2 tbsp chopped fresh parsley

Sprigs of parsley, to garnish

1 Rinse the rice in a sieve (strainer) under cold running water. Cook in a pan of boiling salted water for 12 minutes or according to the packet instructions. Drain well.

2 Meanwhile, trim any fat from the steak and cut into thin strips. Heat the oil in a non-stick frying pan (skillet) and stir-fry the beef for 2 minutes, or until brown and tender. Remove from the pan and set aside.

3 Add the spring onions and pepper to the pan and cook over a high heat, for 3 minutes, stirring, until soft. Sprinkle over the paprika and stir in with salt and pepper to taste.

4 Return the beef to the pan with the crème fraîche and parsley and heat gently for 1 minute until piping hot. Serve on a bed of rice and garnish with sprigs of parsley.

Tuna with Lemon and Coriander

SERVES 2	465 CALORIES PER SERVING
38% CARBOHYDRATE	36% PROTEIN	26% FAT

2 tuna steaks, about 175 g/6 oz each

15 ml/1 tbsp olive oil

Finely grated rind and juice of 1 lemon

15 ml/1 tbsp chopped fresh coriander (cilantro)

Salt and freshly ground black pepper

100 g/4 oz/½ cup long-grain rice

1.2 litres/2 pts/5 cups boiling vegetable stock

1 Put the tuna steaks in a single layer in a shallow dish. Whisk 5 ml/1 tsp oil with the lemon rind and juice. Sprinkle over the steaks, turning them to coat both sides. Cover with clingfilm (plastic wrap) and leave to marinate in the fridge for 2 hours.

2 Heat the remaining oil in a non-stick heavy frying pan (skillet). Remove the tuna from the marinade and cook over a high heat for 2 minutes on each side, then reduce the heat and cook for a further 3 minutes on each side or until cooked through.

3 Add the marinade to the pan and let it bubble for a few seconds, then stir in the chopped fresh coriander. Season to taste with salt and pepper.

4 Meanwhile, cook the rice in the boiling vegetable stock for 10 minutes, or until tender. Drain well. Transfer the tuna to warmed plates. Drizzle over the marinade and serve with the rice.

Poached Salmon and Broccoli with Baked Croûton Topping

SERVES 2		380 CALORIES PER SERVING
50% CARBOHYDRATE	25% PROTEIN	25% FAT

100 g/4 oz broccoli

150 g/5 oz salmon fillet

250 ml/8 fl oz/1 cup skimmed milk

1 bay leaf

20 g/¾ oz/3 tbsp plain (all-purpose) flour

30 ml/2 tbsp chopped fresh dill (dill weed)

3 slices of white bread

Salt and freshly ground black pepper

180 g/6 oz new potatoes

Green salad, to serve

1 Cut the broccoli into small florets and cook in boiling salted water for 3–4 minutes, or until barely tender. Drain well.

2 Meanwhile, put the salmon fillet in a small saucepan with the milk and bay leaf. Slowly bring to the boil and simmer for 3 minutes, or until the fish is just cooked.

3 Remove the fish from the milk and break into chunks, discarding the skin and any bones. Pour the milk into a jug, keeping the bay leaf. Leave to cool.

4 Put the flour in a blender with the milk and mix until smooth. Pour into a small pan, add the bay leaf and bring to the boil, whisking all the time. Simmer for 3 minutes. Remove and discard the bay leaf.

5 Gently mix the salmon, broccoli and dill into the sauce. Season to taste with salt and pepper. Spoon into a flameproof baking dish.

6 Remove the crusts from the bread and cut into small cubes. Sprinkle over the salmon. Cook under a preheated medium grill (broiler) for 3–4 minutes, or until golden brown and crisp. Boil the new potatoes until tender.

7 Serve the salmon with the new potatoes and a crisp green salad.

Blackened Swordfish with Mango Salsa

SERVES 2		460 CALORIES PER SERVING
46% CARBOHYDRATE	40% PROTEIN	14% FAT

2 swordfish steaks, about 175 g/6 oz each

30 ml/2 tbsp plain yoghurt

15 ml/1 tbsp lime juice

2.5 ml/½ tsp ground cumin

2.5 ml/½ tsp ground paprika

2.5 ml/½ tsp dried thyme

A pinch of cayenne

For the Mango Salsa:

1 small ripe mango

½ small red onion

1 red or green chilli, seeded

Juice of ½ lime

10 ml/2 tsp olive oil

Salt and freshly ground black pepper

100 g/4 oz/½ cup long-grain and wild rice

1 Pat the fish dry on kitchen paper (paper towels). Mix together the yoghurt and lime juice and brush over both sides of the fish.

2 Mix the cumin, paprika, thyme and cayenne together and sprinkle over the fish, coating both sides. Set aside in a cool place for 10 minutes.

3 Meanwhile, make the salsa. Peel and dice the mango. Finely chop the red onion and chilli. Add the lime juice, 5 ml/1 tsp olive oil, salt and pepper and mix well. Cover and chill in the fridge until needed.

4 Cook the rice in boiling salted water for 10 minutes, or according to the packet instructions. Drain well and keep warm.

5 Lightly brush a ridged pan or heavy-based frying pan (skillet) with the remaining oil. Heat until very hot. Add the fish and cook for 4 minutes each side, or until cooked through.

6 Serve the swordfish on warmed plates with the rice. Spoon a little of the Mango Salsa on to each plate and serve the rest separately.

Salmon Fillets with Chargrilled Peppers and Dill Couscous

SERVES 2		340 CALORIES PER SERVING
38% CARBOHYDRATE	32% PROTEIN	30% FAT

2 salmon fillets, about 100 g/4 oz each

1 garlic clove, peeled and crushed

5 ml/1 tsp sun-dried tomato purée (paste)

45 ml/3 tbsp plain low-fat yoghurt

Salt and freshly ground black pepper

1 red (bell) pepper

1 yellow pepper

65 g/2½ oz/scant ½ cup couscous

600 ml/1 pt/2½ cups boiling vegetable stock

30 ml/2 tbsp chopped fresh dill (dill weed)

Sprigs of fresh dill, to garnish

1 Put the salmon in a shallow dish. Mix together the garlic, tomato purée, yoghurt, salt and pepper and spread over both sides of the steaks. Cover and marinate in the fridge for 30 minutes.

2 Quarter and seed the peppers, then put them on the grill (broiler) rack, skin-side up. Cook under a preheated grill for 15 minutes, until blistered and charred all over. When cool enough to handle, peel off the skins, then slice.

3 Put the couscous in a bowl and pour over the stock. Leave to soak for 30 minutes, until the grains are soft. Drain off any excess liquid. Stir in the chopped dill and season.

4 Put the salmon on a foil-lined grill rack and cook for about 4 minutes on each side, until firm and the flesh flakes easily when tested with the tip of a knife.

5 Place the grilled salmon on a bed of couscous, topped with the peppers. Garnish with sprigs of fresh dill and serve straight away.

Tip: To make the grilled (broiled) peppers easier to peel, put them in a plastic bag after grilling and seal. After 5 minutes or so, the steam from the heat of the peppers will have loosened the skins.

Plaice and Vegetable Parcels

SERVES 2		285 CALORIES PER SERVING
27% CARBOHYDRATE	43% PROTEIN	30% FAT

15 g/½ oz/1 tbsp butter or polyunsaturated margarine, softened

30 ml/2 tbsp snipped fresh chives

1 small courgette (zucchini), thinly sliced

1 carrot, cut into matchsticks

100 g/4 oz asparagus, trimmed and cut into 2.5 cm/1 in lengths

2 plaice double fillets, about 150 g/5 oz each

4 thin lemon slices

Salt and freshly ground black pepper

175 g/6 oz new potatoes

1 Blend the butter or margarine and chives together. Blanch the courgette, carrot and asparagus in boiling salted water for 1 minute. Drain, reserving the cooking liquid.

2 Cut out two heart shapes from non-stick baking paper, each about 20 × 15 cm/8 × 6 in. Put a plaice fillet, skin-side down, on one side of each heart. Lightly season with salt and pepper. Top each with half of the vegetables and chive butter and two lemon slices.

3 Fold the other side of the paper heart over the fish so that the edges meet. Twist and fold in about 1 cm/½ in of the paper edge all round to make a parcel. Close the parcels by turning the edges of the paper and twisting to secure. Put the parcels on a baking (cookie) sheet.

4 Cook the potatoes in the reserved cooking liquid for 15 minutes or until tender. Meanwhile, bake the fish parcels in a preheated oven at 200°C/400°F/gas mark 6 for 10 minutes.

5 Drain the potatoes and serve on warmed plates with the fish parcels.

Tip: Lemon sole may be used instead of plaice in this recipe, if preferred.

Trout with Toasted Almonds and Cucumber

SERVES 2		440 CALORIES PER SERVING
41% CARBOHYDRATE	29% PROTEIN	30% FAT

½ cucumber

5 ml/1 tsp sunflower oil

2 trout, about 150 g/5 oz each, cleaned and trimmed

25 g/1 oz/¼ cup flaked (slivered) almonds

Salt and freshly ground black pepper

100 g/4 oz/½ cup basmati rice

Lemon wedges, to garnish

1 Cut the cucumber in half lengthways, scoop out the seeds and cut into 5 mm/¼ in thick slices.

2 Brush the oil over the base of a large non-stick frying pan (skillet) over a medium heat. Add the trout and fry (sauté) for about 5 minutes until lightly browned.

3 Turn over the trout and turn down the heat to low. Cook for a further 5 minutes, until cooked through. Remove the trout and keep warm.

4 Turn up the heat and add the cucumber and almonds. Cook until they just begin to turn golden. Season to taste with salt and pepper. Scatter over the fish.

5 Meanwhile, cook the rice in boiling salted water for 10–12 minutes, or until tender. Drain well and serve with the fish, garnished with lemon wedges.

Tip: You can leave the heads on the trout, or remove them, which may make it easier to fit them into the pan.

PASTA, GRAIN AND VEGETARIAN MAIN MEALS

Eating starchy carbohydrates such as pasta, rice and bulgar (cracked) wheat with small helpings of protein is a winning combination from both a nutritional and a slimming point of view. This chapter contains lots of favourite foods such lasagne, pizza and risotto as well as some more unusual recipes. Meatless main courses aren't just for vegetarians and there are plenty of interesting and varied dishes to choose from. In a vegetarian diet, cheese and nuts are good sources of protein and are often the mainstays of meat-free meals. However, they're also high in fat and calories and should be eaten sparingly. Pulses and beans are protein-packed, especially when teamed with grains. If you're vegetarian, make sure that you get enough iron. Eating or drinking vitamin-C-rich foods – like a small glass of orange juice – with a meal helps the body to absorb iron. Tea or coffee can inhibit iron absorption, so avoid these drinks for at least half an hour before and after eating.

Tagliatelle with Creamy Spinach Sauce

SERVES 2		425 CALORIES PER SERVING
68% CARBOHYDRATE	14% PROTEIN	18% FAT

175 g/6 oz young leaf spinach

50 g/2 oz Gorgonzola cheese

30 ml/2 tbsp skimmed milk

Freshly ground black pepper

175 g/6 oz tagliatelle

A pinch of salt

1 Wash the spinach and remove any tough stalks. Put in a pan and gently cook for 2–3 minutes until just wilted. Remove from the heat and drain.

2 Chop the Gorgonzola and put in a small pan with the milk. Heat gently until melted, stirring occasionally. Stir in the wilted spinach and season to taste with black pepper.

3 Cook the pasta in plenty of boiling salted water for 10 minutes or until *al dente*. Drain, then add the spinach sauce and gently mix together. Serve straight away.

Smoked Salmon and Dill Fettucine

SERVES 3		385 CALORIES PER SERVING
65% CARBOHYDRATE	18% PROTEIN	17% FAT

225 g/8 oz fresh green and white fettucine

A pinch of salt

75 g/3 oz/⅓ cup curd (smooth cottage) cheese

75 ml/5 tbsp half-fat crème fraîche

75 g/3 oz smoked salmon trimmings

45 ml/3 tbsp chopped fresh dill (dill weed)

Freshly ground black pepper

Lemon wedges and sprigs of fresh dill, to garnish

1 Cook the fettucine in plenty of boiling salted water for 2–3 minutes, or according to the packet instructions. Drain.

2 Meanwhile, gently heat the curd cheese and crème fraîche until melted. Cut the smoked salmon into small strips and stir into the sauce with the chopped dill. Season with pepper.

3 Add the sauce to the fettucine and gently toss together. Serve hot, garnished with lemon wedges and sprigs of fresh dill.

Warm Pasta Salad

SERVES 2	390 CALORIES PER SERVING
71% CARBOHYDRATE	22% PROTEIN	7% FAT

1 red (bell) pepper, quartered

1 green pepper, quartered

175 g/6 oz dried fusilli

100 g/3½ oz/1 small can of tuna in brine, drained and flaked

45 ml/3 tbsp no-fat Greek yoghurt

Salt and freshly ground black pepper

Mixed salad, to serve

1 Place the peppers on a grill (broiler) pan, skin-side up. Grill (broil) for 5–6 minutes or until the skins are blackened and charred in places.

2 Put the peppers in a plastic bag or a bowl covered with clingfilm (plastic wrap) and leave until cool. When cold, peel off the skins and discard. Slice the peppers.

3 Meanwhile, cook the pasta in boiling salted water for 10 minutes or until tender but still with a little 'bite'. Drain thoroughly.

4 Put the warm pasta in a bowl with the peppers, flaked tuna and yoghurt. Season to taste with salt and pepper and serve straight away with a large mixed salad.

Spaghetti Leonardo

SERVES 2		340 CALORIES PER SERVING
47% CARBOHYDRATE	23% PROTEIN	30% FAT

100 g/4 oz spaghetti

10 ml/2 tsp olive oil

50 g/2 oz button mushrooms, halved

50 g/2 oz/¼ cup half-fat cream cheese

225 g/8 oz fresh baby spinach

50 g/2 oz Parma ham, cut into slivers

Salt and freshly ground black pepper

15 ml/1 tbsp freshly grated Parmesan cheese

1 Cook the spaghetti in boiling salted water for 10 minutes, or according to the packet instructions. Drain thoroughly.

2 Meanwhile, heat the oil in a heavy-based non-stick frying pan (skillet) and gently cook the mushrooms for 4–5 minutes, until soft. Add the half-fat cream cheese and stir until melted.

3 Add the mushroom mixture, spinach and Parma ham to the hot spaghetti and season with salt and pepper. Toss together, so that the sauce coats the spaghetti and the spinach starts to wilt.

4 Spoon the spaghetti on to warmed plates and serve straight away, sprinkled with Parmesan.

Marinated Tofu and Noodle Stir-fry

SERVES 2		325 CALORIES PER SERVING	
54% CARBOHYDRATE	19% PROTEIN	25% FAT	2% ALCOHOL

5 ml/1 tsp sesame oil

15 ml/1 tbsp dark soy sauce

15 ml/1 tbsp dry sherry

100 g/4 oz firm tofu, cut into cubes

100 g/4 oz Chinese egg noodles

15 ml/1 tbsp sunflower oil

1 bunch of spring onions (scallions), trimmed and diagonally sliced

1 carrot, thinly sliced

2.5 cm/1 in piece of root ginger, peeled and finely grated

1 garlic clove, peeled and crushed

50 g/2 oz button mushrooms, sliced

100 g/4 oz broccoli, trimmed and divided into tiny florets

120 ml/4 fl oz/½ cup vegetable stock

10 ml/2 tsp cornflour (cornstarch)

1 Mix the sesame oil, soy sauce and sherry together in a shallow bowl. Add the tofu, toss to coat and leave to marinate for 30 minutes.

2 Cook the noodles in plenty of boiling water according to the packet instructions. Drain well and set aside.

3 Heat the sunflower oil in a wok or large frying pan (skillet) over a high heat. Add the spring onions, carrot and ginger and stir-fry for 3 minutes.

4 Add the garlic, mushrooms and broccoli, cook for 1 minute, then pour in half the stock. Lower the heat, cover and simmer for 3 minutes.

5 Put the cornflour in a small bowl, and pour in the marinade from the tofu. Blend to a paste, then stir into the remaining stock. Add to the wok and cook, stirring all the time, until thickened.

6 Add the tofu and noodles to the pan and gently mix with the vegetables. Gently heat for a minute or two until piping hot. Serve straight away.

Spiced Coconut Couscous

SERVES 2		240 CALORIES PER SERVING
56% CARBOHYDRATE	14% PROTEIN	30% FAT

100 g/4 oz/⅔ cup couscous

5 ml/1 tsp olive oil

1 garlic clove, peeled and finely chopped

4 spring onions (scallions), trimmed and sliced

2.5 ml/½ tsp ground coriander (cilantro)

2.5 ml/½ tsp ground cumin

1 red chilli, seeded and finely chopped

1 medium courgette (zucchini)

1 small aubergine (eggplant)

350 ml/12 fl oz/1½ cups vegetable stock

15 ml/1 tbsp lemon juice

15 g/½ oz creamed coconut, finely chopped

A pinch of saffron strands

75 g/3 oz drained canned chick peas (garbanzos)

15 ml/1 tbsp chopped fresh coriander or parsley

15 ml/1 tbsp chopped fresh mint

Salt and freshly ground pepper

Sprigs of fresh coriander (cilantro), parsley or mint, to garnish

1 Moisten the couscous according to the packet instructions. Heat the oil in a non-stick saucepan over which a steamer, metal sieve (strainer) or colander will fit. Add the garlic, spring onions, ground coriander, cumin and chilli and cook for a minute, stirring.

2 Cut the courgette and aubergine into 2 cm/¾ in chunks. Add to the pan with the stock, lemon juice, coconut and saffron. Bring to the boil and gently simmer, uncovered, for 8 minutes. Stir in the chick peas.

3 Meanwhile, fork the couscous to separate the grains and spoon into the steamer lined with muslin (cheesecloth) or a clean J-cloth. Place over the vegetables. Cover and cook for 5 minutes or until the couscous is hot and the vegetables tender.

4 Stir the chopped fresh herbs into the vegetables, then season to taste with salt and pepper. Spoon the couscous on to warmed plates and top with the vegetables. Serve garnished with sprigs of coriander, parsley or mint.

Fresh Asparagus and Pine Nut Risotto

SERVES 2		465 CALORIES PER SERVING
61% CARBOHYDRATE	12% PROTEIN	25% FAT	4% ALCOHOL

100 g/4 oz fresh asparagus tips, trimmed

15 ml/1 tbsp olive oil

1 small onion, finely chopped

175 g/6 oz/⅔ cup risotto (arborio) rice

A pinch of saffron strands (optional)

60 ml/4 tbsp dry white wine

350 ml/12 fl oz/1½ cups boiling vegetable stock

Juice and rind of ½ lemon

Salt and freshly ground black pepper

30 ml/2 tbsp pine nuts, toasted

15 ml/1 tbsp grated Parmesan cheese

1 Blanch the asparagus in boiling salted water for 3 minutes, or until almost tender. Drain and refresh immediately under cold running water.

2 Heat the oil in a heavy-based pan and gently cook the onion for 4 minutes or until beginning to soften. Stir in the rice and saffron, if using, and cook for 1 minute.

3 Add the wine, stock, lemon rind, 15 ml/1 tbsp lemon juice, the salt and pepper. Bring to the boil, stirring. Cover and simmer for 8 minutes.

4 Carefully stir in the asparagus and cook for a further 2 minutes, or until the rice is tender and most of the liquid absorbed.

5 Remove the lemon rind and stir in the pine nuts. Spoon on to warmed plates and serve with shavings of Parmesan cheese.

Bulgar Wheat with Feta and Mint

SERVES 2		450 CALORIES PER SERVING
55% CARBOHYDRATE	18% PROTEIN	27% FAT

150 g/5 oz/scant 1 cup bulgar (cracked) wheat

150 ml/¼ pint/⅔ cup boiling vegetable stock

½ cucumber, chopped

4 spring onions (scallions), trimmed and sliced

4 tomatoes, skinned, seeded and chopped

15 ml/1 tbsp chopped fresh mint

15 ml/1 tbsp olive oil

15 ml/1 tbsp lemon juice

Salt and freshly ground black pepper

75 g/3 oz/scant ⅓ cup Feta cheese, diced

Sprigs of fresh mint, to garnish

1 Put the bulgar wheat in a bowl and pour over the vegetable stock. Leave for 30 minutes, stirring occasionally, until the water has been absorbed.

2 Stir in the cucumber, spring onions, tomatoes and mint. Whisk together the oil and lemon juice and stir in. Season to taste with salt and pepper. Cover and chill in the fridge for at least 30 minutes.

3 Stir the Feta cheese into the bulgar. Spoon on to individual plates and serve each garnished with a sprig of mint.

Vegetable Cassoulet

SERVES 2   465 CALORIES PER SERVING

68% CARBOHYDRATE   20% PROTEIN   12% FAT

10 ml/2 tsp olive oil

1 onion, finely chopped

1 garlic clove, peeled and crushed

1 leek, thickly sliced

2 carrots, sliced

150 ml/¼ pt/⅔ cup vegetable stock

1 bay leaf

200 g/7 oz/1 small can of chopped tomatoes

10 ml/2 tsp tomato purée (paste)

425 g/15 oz/1 large can of haricot beans or mixed pulses

10 ml/2 tsp chopped fresh thyme

15 ml/1 tbsp chopped fresh parsley

Salt and freshly ground black pepper

75 g/3 oz/1½ cups fresh white breadcrumbs

1 Heat the oil in a flameproof casserole (Dutch oven) and gently cook the onion and garlic for 10 minutes or until soft. Add the leek, carrots, stock, bay leaf, tomatoes and tomato purée.

2 Bring to the boil, cover and simmer for 10 minutes. Stir in the beans and their liquid, the thyme, parsley, salt and pepper.

3 Sprinkle the top with breadcrumbs and bake, uncovered, in a preheated oven at 160°C/325°F/gas mark 3 for 30 minutes, or until the topping is golden brown and crisp and the vegetables tender.

Baked Butternut Squash with Red Pesto and Bean Stuffing

SERVES 2		265 CALORIES PER SERVING
50% CARBOHYDRATE	20% PROTEIN	30% FAT

350 g/12 oz butternut squash

2.5 ml/½ tsp paprika

150 g/5 oz/1 small can of mixed pulses

2 tomatoes, seeded and chopped

30 ml/2 tbsp red pesto

15 ml/1 tbsp lemon juice

Salt and freshly ground black pepper

15 g/½ oz/¼ cup fresh white breadcrumbs

15 ml/1 tbsp freshly grated mature Cheddar cheese

1 Cut the butternut squash in half lengthways. Scoop out the seeds and discard. Score the cut surface in a criss-cross fashion with a sharp knife and sprinkle with paprika.

2 For the stuffing, drain the can of pulses and put in a bowl with the tomatoes, pesto, lemon juice, salt and pepper. Mix together well and spoon into the hollows of the squash.

3 Mix together the breadcrumbs and cheese and sprinkle over the stuffing. Put the squash halves in a roasting tin (pan). Pour 150 ml/¼ pt/⅔ cup hot water around the squash and cover the tin with foil.

4 Bake at 180°C/350°F/gas mark 4 for 45 minutes. Remove the foil and cook for a further 15 minutes, or until the squash is very tender and the topping browned. Serve hot.

Upside-down Pizza

SERVES 2		340 CALORIES PER SERVING
55% CARBOHYDRATE	16% PROTEIN	29% FAT

1 large tomato, thinly sliced

½ green or yellow (bell) pepper, thinly sliced

25 g/1 oz sliced pepperoni stick

25 g/1 oz stoned (pitted) black olives in brine, halved

50 g/2 oz/½ cup plain (all-purpose) flour

50 g/2 oz/½ cup plain wholemeal flour

2.5 ml/½ tsp baking powder

1.5 ml/¼ tsp salt

2.5 ml/½ tsp dried mixed herbs

15 g/½ oz/2 tbsp butter or polyunsaturated margarine

About 75 ml/5 tbsp skimmed milk

Mixed salad, to serve

1 Arrange the tomato and pepper slices with the pepperoni and black olives on the base of a lightly greased non-stick 18 cm/7 in round shallow cake tin (pan).

2 Put the flours, baking powder, salt and herbs in a mixing bowl. Rub in the butter or margarine until the mixture resembles fine breadcrumbs. Stir in enough milk to make a fairly soft dough.

3 On a lightly floured surface, roll out the dough to fit the tin and place on top of the vegetables and salami. Bake in a preheated oven at 200°C/400°F/gas mark 6 for 20 minutes, or until well risen and golden brown.

4 Turn out the pizza and cut into four wedges. Serve hot with a mixed salad.

Vegetable Platter with Chilli and Coriander Chutney

SERVES 2		265 CALORIES PER SERVING
48% CARBOHYDRATE	22% PROTEIN	30% FAT

For the Chilli and Coriander Chutney:

4 tomatoes

1 small red onion

3 red chillis

Juice of 1 lime

10 ml/2 tsp olive oil

30 ml/2 tbsp chopped fresh coriander (cilantro)

For the Vegetable Platter:

350 g/12 oz small courgettes (zucchini)

1 medium aubergine (eggplant), about 300 g/10 oz

1 red (bell) pepper

10 ml/2 tsp olive oil

Salt and freshly ground black pepper

2 slices of white bread, crusts removed

50 g/2 oz reduced-fat (light) Mozzarella cheese

1 First, make the chutney. Skin, seed and chop the tomatoes. Peel and finely chop the onion. Halve, seed and finely chop the red chillis. Put in a bowl with the lime juice, olive oil and coriander and mix together. Cover and chill until ready to serve.

2 Trim the courgettes and slice into 5 mm/¼ in rounds. Cut the aubergine into 1 cm/½ in rounds, then cut each round into quarters. Halve and seed the pepper. Cut each half into four strips.

3 Put the vegetables on a grill (broiler) pan and sprinkle with the oil and a little salt and pepper. Cook under a hot grill for 10–15 minutes, turning several times, until lightly browned and tender.

4 Meanwhile, cut the bread and Mozzarella into 1 cm/½ in cubes. Scatter over the vegetables and return to the grill for a further minute or until the bread is toasted and the cheese beginning to melt. Transfer to warmed plates and serve with the chutney.

Grilled Porcini Polenta with Red Onion Gravy

SERVES 2		385 CALORIES PER SERVING	
50% CARBOHYDRATE	14% PROTEIN	23% FAT	13% ALCOHOL

15 g/½ oz packet of dried porcini mushrooms

100 g/4 oz/1 cup instant polenta (cornmeal)

25 g/1 oz/¼ cup grated Parmesan

15 ml/1 tbsp chopped fresh parsley

Salt and freshly ground black pepper

For the Red Onion Gravy:

10 ml/2 tsp olive oil

1 red onion, thinly sliced

150 ml/¼ pt/⅔ cup red wine

150 ml/¼ pt/⅔ cup vegetable stock

15 ml/1 tbsp plain (all-purpose) flour, for dusting

A little extra olive oil, for frying (sautéing)

1 Put the mushrooms in a bowl and pour over 150 ml/ ¼ pt/⅔ cup boiling water. Leave to soak for 30 minutes, then drain, reserving the soaking liquid.

2 Meanwhile, bring 500 ml/17 fl oz/2¼ cups water to the boil. Add the polenta in a steady stream, stirring all the time. Simmer for 10 minutes, or according to the packet instructions. Stir in the Parmesan, parsley, salt and pepper.

3 Pour into a shallow 18 cm/7 in square non-stick baking tin (pan), base-lined with non-stick baking parchment and leave to cool and set.

4 Meanwhile, make the Red Onion Gravy. Heat the oil in a heavy non-stick frying pan (skillet). Add the onion and gently cook for 10 minutes, or until soft. Pour in the wine, stock and soaking liquid from the mushrooms. Simmer until reduced by half. Season with salt and pepper.

5 Turn out the polenta and cut into squares. Dust each with a little flour. Brush a non-stick frying pan with a little oil and heat until smoking hot. Sear the polenta for 1–2 minutes on each side. Serve with the Red Onion Gravy.

Jerusalem Artichoke and Tomato Gratin

SERVES 2		175 CALORIES PER SERVING
69% CARBOHYDRATE	12% PROTEIN	19% FAT

350 g/12 oz Jerusalem artichokes

30 ml/2 tbsp red wine vinegar

4 large red or yellow tomatoes

10 ml/2 tsp olive oil

2.5 ml/½ tsp wholegrain mustard

1 garlic clove, peeled and crushed

15 ml/1 tbsp snipped fresh chives

Salt and freshly ground black pepper

25 g/1 oz/½ cup fresh white breadcrumbs

1 Peel the artichokes and drop them into a bowl of cold water with 5 ml/1 tsp vinegar, to prevent them turning brown. Stir 15 ml/1 tbsp vinegar into a pan of boiling salted water.

2 Add the artichokes to the boiling water and cook for 8 minutes or until barely tender. Drain and cool.

3 Meanwhile, slice the tomatoes. Mix the oil, the remaining 10 ml/2 tsp vinegar, the mustard, garlic and chives together and season with salt and pepper. Slice the artichokes and immediately toss in the mixture to coat.

4 Arrange the tomato and artichoke slices in a 900 ml/ 1½ pt/3¾ cup ovenproof dish, overlapping them slightly. Sprinkle over the breadcrumbs.

5 Bake the gratin in a preheated oven at 180°C/350°F/gas mark 4 for 30 minutes, or until the topping is lightly browned and crisp. Serve straight away.

VEGETABLES AND SALADS

Juicy, red, ripe tomatoes or tender, young, green spears of asparagus: vegetable accompaniments like these can be an appetising and colourful part of your main meal. Not only are they delicious, they also play an important part in a healthy diet, providing lots of fibre and vitamins. They're low in calories too, as long as you don't toss them in butter, cream or a rich dressing. Take a look at the salads in this section when planning your daily menu. Many of them can be served as a light meal. And don't reserve salads just for the summer months; supermarkets stock a huge range of salad ingredients all year round. Try a hot salad for a change, such as Goats' Cheese and Chive Croûton Salad (page 113) or Warm Prawn and Feta with Spinach (page 117). Try to eat several helpings of cooked or raw vegetables and fruit each day and add variety by choosing different flavours, colours and textures.

Mixed Mushroom Sauté

SERVES 2		60 CALORIES PER SERVING
25% CARBOHYDRATE	30% PROTEIN	11% FAT 34% ALCOHOL

1 small onion, finely chopped

1 garlic clove, finely chopped

60 ml/4 tbsp dry red wine

100 ml/3½ fl oz/scant ½ cup vegetable stock

15 ml/1 tbsp light soy sauce

5 ml/1 tsp chopped fresh thyme

225 g/8 oz mixed mushrooms, halved or sliced if large

10 ml/2 tsp wine vinegar

30 ml/2 tbsp chopped fresh parsley

Salt and freshly ground black pepper

1   Put the onion, garlic, wine, stock and soy sauce in a saucepan. Cover and simmer for 5 minutes. Uncover and simmer for 5 more minutes, until there is only about 45 ml/3 tbsp liquid left.

2   Add the thyme, mushrooms and vinegar and continue cooking for a further 5–6 minutes until the mushrooms are cooked, but still firm.

3   Stir in the parsley, then season the mushrooms to taste with salt and pepper. Remove from the heat and serve straight away.

Tip: Use a selection of mushrooms such as chestnut, shiitake, ceps, girolles and oyster mushrooms.

Spiced Broccoli with Balsamic Vinegar

SERVES 2		150 CALORIES PER SERVING
50% CARBOHYDRATE	20% PROTEIN	30% FAT

350 g/12 oz broccoli

40 g/1½ oz/⅓ cup quick-cook polenta (cornmeal)

5 ml/1 tsp cumin seeds, lightly crushed

1.5 ml/¼ tsp ground turmeric

Salt and freshly ground black pepper

10 ml/2 tsp olive oil

1 small onion, thinly sliced

15 ml/1 tbsp balsamic vinegar

1 Cut the broccoli into florets. Add to a pan of boiling salted water and cook for 1 minute. Drain and refresh in cold water, then drain again.

2 Mix together the polenta, cumin and turmeric and season with salt and pepper. Add the blanched broccoli florets and mix together until coated.

3 Heat the oil in a non-stick frying pan (skillet). Add the onion and cook gently for 4 minutes. Add the broccoli and cook for a further 4–5 minutes until crisp and tender. Sprinkle with the vinegar and serve straight away.

Candied Sweet Potato with Orange

SERVES 2		190 CALORIES PER SERVING
67% CARBOHYDRATE	4% PROTEIN	29% FAT

225 g/8 oz sweet potatoes

5 ml/1 tsp groundnut (peanut) or sunflower oil

5 ml/1 tsp unsalted butter

30 ml/2 tbsp orange juice

2.5 ml/½ tsp finely grated orange rind

10 ml/2 tsp demerara sugar

Salt and freshly ground black pepper

1 Peel the sweet potatoes and cut into 5 cm/2 in chunks. Put the oil and butter in a small non-stick roasting tin (pan) and put in a preheated oven at 200°C/400°F/gas mark 6 for 2–3 minutes.

2 Add the sweet potatoes to the pan, turning them to coat. Cook in the oven for 45 minutes, turning occasionally.

3 Mix together the orange juice and rind, sugar, salt and pepper. Drizzle over the potatoes and cook for a further 15–20 minutes, until caramelised and tender.

Goats' Cheese and Chive Croûton Salad

SERVES 2		345 CALORIES PER SERVING
54% CARBOHYDRATE	16% PROTEIN	30% FAT

1 small French baguette

75 g/3 oz firm round goats' cheese

10 ml/2 tsp walnut oil

5 ml/1 tsp white wine vinegar

2.5 ml/½ tsp Dijon mustard

15 ml/1 tbsp snipped fresh chives

Salt and freshly ground black pepper

100 g/4 oz mixed salad leaves, eg rocket (arugula), oak leaf and lambs' lettuce

1 Cut the baguette into six slices and arrange on a baking (cookie) tray. Cut the cheese into six thin slices and put on top of the bread.

2 Bake in a preheated oven at 190°C/375°F/gas mark 5 for 10 minutes, or until the cheese has just begun to melt.

3 Put the oil, vinegar, mustard and chives in a small bowl and whisk with a fork to combine. Season to taste with salt and pepper.

4 Arrange the salad leaves on two plates and drizzle over the dressing. Top with the cheese croûtons and serve straight away.

Chargrilled Aubergines with Lemon Vinaigrette

SERVES 2		160 CALORIES PER SERVING
66% CARBOHYDRATE	11% PROTEIN	23% FAT

1 medium aubergine (eggplant)

1.5 ml/¼ tsp salt

30 ml/2 tbsp olive oil

Juice of 1 lemon

15 ml/1 tbsp soft light brown sugar

A few torn basil leaves, to garnish

2 slices of crusty bread, to serve

1 Cut the aubergine lengthways into 1.25 cm/½ in slices and season with a little salt. Leave for 5 minutes, then pat dry on kitchen paper (paper towels). Lightly brush both sides with olive oil.

2 Heat a ridged griddle pan or heavy-based non-stick frying pan (skillet). Add the aubergine slices, then sprinkle with half the lemon juice and sugar. Cook over a medium heat for 3–4 minutes until lightly browned.

3 Turn the aubergine slices over and sprinkle with the remaining lemon juice and sugar. Cook for a further 3–4 minutes until tender and caramelised. Scatter with torn basil leaves and serve with slices of crusty bread.

Pesto Potatoes

SERVES 4		135 CALORIES PER SERVING
57% CARBOHYDRATE	13% PROTEIN	30% FAT

450 g/1 lb small new potatoes

1 garlic clove, peeled and crushed

15 g/½ oz fresh basil leaves

15 g/½ oz/2 tbsp pine nuts

10 ml/2 tsp olive oil

45 ml/3 tbsp no-fat Greek yoghurt

Salt and freshly ground black pepper

4 spring onions (scallions), trimmed and thinly sliced

A sprig of fresh basil, to garnish

1 Cook the potatoes in boiling salted water for 15 minutes or until just tender. Drain well.

2 Meanwhile, make the pesto. Put the garlic, basil, pine nuts, oil and yoghurt in a blender or food processor. Season with a little salt and pepper. Blend until fairly smooth.

3 Put the hot potatoes in a warmed serving dish with the spring onions. Pour over the pesto sauce and toss to coat. Serve garnished with a sprig of basil.

Celery and Chicory Braise

SERVES 2		40 CALORIES PER SERVING
76% CARBOHYDRATE	12% PROTEIN	12% FAT

1 head of chicory (Belgian endive)

5 ml/1 tsp chopped fresh thyme

Salt and freshly ground black pepper

2 celery sticks

1 orange

1 lime

1 Cut the chicory into quarters lengthways and put in an ovenproof dish, cut side down. Sprinkle with the thyme and season with salt and pepper.

2 Cut the celery sticks in half, then cut into long thin slices. Put on top of the chicory.

3 Finely grate the rind of half the orange, then squeeze the juice from the orange and lime. Pour over the vegetables.

4 Cover with a lid or foil and cook in a preheated oven at 190°C/375°F/gas mark 4 for 25–30 minutes or until tender.

Warm Prawn and Feta with Spinach

SERVES 2		325 CALORIES PER SERVING
38% CARBOHYDRATE	32% PROTEIN	30% FAT

100 g/4 oz baby spinach leaves

75 g/3 oz/⅓ cup Feta cheese

15 ml/1 tbsp olive oil

10 ml/2 tsp chopped fresh oregano or marjoram

175 g/6 oz uncooked large prawns (jumbo shrimp), shelled and veins removed

15 ml/1 tbsp lemon juice

Salt and freshly ground black pepper

2 crusty wholemeal rolls

1 Arrange the spinach on two plates. Cut the Feta cheese into 1 cm/½ in cubes. Toss in 5 ml/1 tsp oil, then sprinkle with the oregano or marjoram and toss again to coat.

2 Heat the remaining oil in a non-stick frying pan (skillet). Add the prawns and cook for 1–2 minutes on each side until pink and cooked through. Add the cheese and stir for a few seconds until beginning to melt.

3 Sprinkle over the lemon juice and spoon on top of the spinach. Season with salt and pepper to taste before serving with crusty wholemeal rolls.

Hot Potato Salad

SERVES 2	225 CALORIES PER SERVING

52% CARBOHYDRATE	18% PROTEIN	30% FAT

350 g/12 oz new potatoes

15 ml/1 tbsp light olive oil

2 rashers (slices) of lean back bacon, chopped

2 celery sticks, chopped

5 ml/1 tsp Dijon mustard

15 ml/1 tbsp lemon juice

10 ml/2 tsp capers, drained

Salt and freshly ground black pepper

A few chopped celery leaves, to garnish

1 Scrub the potatoes and cook in boiling salted water for 15 minutes or until tender. Drain and cut into 2.5 cm/ 1 in chunks. Put in a warmed serving dish.

2 Meanwhile, make the dressing. Heat the oil in a frying pan (skillet) and cook the bacon until crisp. Remove and set aside. Add the celery and cook gently for 5 minutes until soft.

3 Return the bacon to the pan with the mustard, lemon juice and capers and season with salt and pepper. Add to the hot potatoes and mix well. Serve sprinkled with chopped celery leaves.

Marinated Cucumber and Dill Salad

SERVES 4   80 CALORIES PER SERVING

79% CARBOHYDRATE   6% PROTEIN   2% FAT   13% ALCOHOL

2 medium cucumbers

15 ml/1 tbsp salt

50 g/2 oz/¼ cup granulated sugar

150 ml/¼ pt/⅔ cup dry cider

15 ml/1 tbsp cider vinegar

30 ml/2 tbsp chopped fresh dill (dill weed)

1 Slice the cucumbers as thinly as possible and place in a colander, lightly sprinkling salt between the layers. Put the colander over a bowl and leave to drain for 30 minutes.

2 Rinse the cucumber slices under cold running water to remove the salt, then pat them dry with kitchen paper (paper towels).

3 Put the sugar in a small pan with the cider. Heat very gently until the sugar dissolves. Remove from the heat and leave until tepid. Stir in the cider vinegar. Add the cucumber slices, cover and leave for 2–3 hours.

4 Drain the cucumber, discarding the marinade. Add the dill to the cucumber and mix well. Turn into a serving dish, cover with clingfilm (plastic wrap) and chill in the fridge until needed.

Italian Country Salad

SERVES 2		250 CALORIES PER SERVING
50% CARBOHYDRATE	20% PROTEIN	30% FAT

100 g/4 oz fine green beans

100 g/4 oz small courgettes (zucchini)

1 garlic clove, peeled and crushed

10 ml/2 tsp red wine vinegar

10 ml/2 tsp olive oil

Salt and freshly ground black pepper

4 ripe tomatoes, skinned, seeded and chopped

200 g/7 oz/1 medium can of artichoke hearts in brine, drained

25 g/1 oz stoned (pitted) black olives, in brine

15 g/½ oz Parmesan cheese

2 slices of ciabatta bread, to serve

1 Wash and trim the beans and slice the courgettes. Cook the beans in boiling salted water for 2 minutes. Add the courgettes and cook for 1–2 minutes or until tender. Drain thoroughly.

2 Mix together the garlic, vinegar and oil, and season with salt and pepper. Stir in the tomatoes. Put the beans, courgettes, artichokes and olives in a bowl. Pour over the dressing and toss together to mix.

3 Cut the Parmesan into thin slivers with a potato peeler and scatter over the salad. Serve straight away, accompanied with a slice of plain or toasted ciabatta for each person.

Tip: Use 100 g/4 oz red or yellow cherry tomatoes instead of the chopped tomatoes, if preferred.

Gingered Carrot, Nut and Raisin Salad

SERVES 2		140 CALORIES PER SERVING
68% CARBOHYDRATE	6% PROTEIN	26% FAT

50 g/2 oz/⅓ cup raisins

30 ml/2 tbsp orange juice

225 g/8 oz carrots

15 g/½ oz/1 tbsp skinned toasted hazelnuts (filberts), chopped

5 ml/1 tsp grated fresh root ginger

10 ml/2 tsp hazelnut or sunflower oil

Salt and freshly ground black pepper

1 Put the raisins in a bowl with the orange juice and leave to soak for at least 30 minutes, to plump up the fruit.

2 Peel and coarsely grate the carrots. Put in a bowl with the hazelnuts and ginger.

3 Stir the oil into the raisins. Add to the carrots and season to taste with salt and pepper. Mix well and turn into a serving bowl.

Sweet and Sour Red Salad

SERVES 2		140 CALORIES PER SERVING
60% CARBOHYDRATE	10% PROTEIN	30% FAT

225 g/8 oz red cabbage

1 red onion

1 red (bell) pepper

100 g/4 oz cooked beetroot (red beets)

10 ml/2 tsp sesame oil

5 ml/1 tsp red wine vinegar

10 ml/2 tsp clear honey

10 ml/2 tsp light soy sauce

Salt and freshly ground black pepper

1 Remove the core from the cabbage, then finely shred. Finely slice the red onion and pepper and cut the beetroot into matchsticks. Put in a bowl and mix together.

2 For the dressing, put the oil, vinegar, honey and soy sauce in a jug. Season with salt and pepper and whisk together with a fork.

3 Pour the dressing over the vegetables and toss well to mix. Cover and leave to stand for 2–3 hours before serving to allow the flavours to mingle.

Pear and Blue Cheese Salad

SERVES 2		340 CALORIES PER SERVING
55% CARBOHYDRATE	15% PROTEIN	30% FAT

25 g/1 oz Stilton or Roquefort cheese

15 ml/1 tbsp walnut oil

15 g/½ oz/1 tbsp walnut pieces

2 small ripe pears

15 ml/1 tbsp lemon juice

6 large radicchio leaves

Salt and freshly ground black pepper

2 crusty wholemeal rolls, to serve

1 Remove the rind from the cheese and crumble into small pieces. Heat the oil in a pan and gently cook the walnuts for 2–3 minutes until lightly toasted.

2 Quarter and core the pears. Thinly peel, if liked, then cut into thin slices and toss in the lemon juice to prevent them from going brown.

3 Tear the radicchio leaves in half and arrange them on two plates. Add the walnuts and blue cheese to the pear slices and season with salt and pepper. Divide the mixture between the plates and serve straight away with crusty wholemeal rolls.

LOW-FAT DESSERTS

Ices, jellies, tarts and puddings make a
happy ending to any meal and you
don't have to miss out if you're on a
diet. In this section, there are more than
a dozen delectable desserts, not one of
them containing more than 250 calories
and most much less. Many make the
most of fresh fruit or low-fat yoghurt,
but there are also more sumptuous
desserts, such as Dark Chocolate Soufflés
(page 134), that will appeal to dieters
and non-dieters alike. Others, such as
Autumn Pudding (page 140) are perfect
for party entertaining.
When serving puddings, avoid cream
and stick to moderate helpings of
accompaniments such as yoghurt,
fromage frais and low-fat custard or
ice-cream.

Sparkling Orange Jellies with Minted Crème Fraîche

SERVES 2	200 CALORIES PER SERVING

60% CARBOHYDRATE	8.5% PROTEIN	30% FAT	1.5% ALCOHOL

250 ml/8 fl oz/1 cup fresh orange juice

7.5 ml/1½ tsp powdered gelatine

1 orange

50 g/2 oz small seedless grapes, halved

100 ml/3½ fl oz/scant ½ cup half-fat crème fraîche

10 ml/2 tsp icing (confectioners') sugar, sifted

15 ml/1 tbsp chopped fresh mint

5 ml/1 tsp crème de menthe liqueur (optional)

1 Pour 60 ml/4 tbsp orange juice into a small heatproof bowl, sprinkle on the gelatine and leave to soak for 5 minutes. Put the bowl over a pan of near-boiling water and stir until dissolved. Leave until cool, then stir into the remaining orange juice.

2 With a sharp knife, peel the orange and remove all the white pith. Remove the segments by cutting between the membranes.

3 Divide the orange segments and grapes between two sundae glasses. Pour in enough orange jelly (jello) to cover the fruit and chill until just set. Pour on the remaining orange jelly and chill for a further 3–4 hours until set.

4 For the minted crème fraîche, mix the crème fraîche, icing sugar, mint and liqueur together and spoon into a small bowl. Chill.

5 Serve the jellies with the Minted Crème Fraîche spooned over the top.

Peach Yoghurt Brûlée

SERVES 2	125 CALORIES PER SERVING
72.5% CARBOHYDRATE	27% PROTEIN 0.5% FAT

2 ripe peaches or nectarines, halved, stoned (pitted)
and sliced

150 g/5 oz/1 small carton of no-fat Greek yoghurt

5 ml/1 tsp vanilla esssence (extract)

30 ml/2 tbsp demerara sugar

1   Arrange the fruit in the base of two small individual flameproof dishes. Mix the Greek yoghurt and vanilla essence together and spoon over the fruit, smoothing the surface with the back of the spoon.

2   Sprinkle the sugar evenly over the top to cover the yoghurt completely – use a little extra, if needed.

3   Cook under a preheated grill (broiler) for about 1 minute or until the sugar has melted. Chill in the fridge for 30 minutes before serving.

Fresh Fruit with Golden Glazed Sabayon

SERVES 2		190 CALORIES PER SERVING	
59% CARBOHYDRATE	10% PROTEIN	27% FAT	4% ALCOHOL

350 g/12 oz mixed summer fruits, eg strawberries, raspberries, blueberries and cherries

15 ml/1 tbsp kirsch

2 egg yolks

25 g/1 oz/2 tbsp caster (superfine) sugar

10 ml/2 tsp icing (confectioners') sugar

1 Prepare the fruit and toss in a bowl with the kirsch. Divide between two shallow, flameproof dishes.

2 Put the egg yolks and caster sugar in a bowl over a pan of barely simmering water and whisk for 6–8 minutes or until the mixture is very thick and pale.

3 Spoon the whisked mixture over the fruit. Cook under a preheated medium grill (broiler) for 2–3 minutes or until dark golden. Dust with icing sugar and serve straight away.

Red Fruit Fool

SERVES 2	75 CALORIES PER SERVING

61% CARBOHYDRATE	35% PROTEIN	4% FAT

225 g/8 oz mixed red fruit, such as raspberries, redcurrants, cherries and strawberries

10 ml/2 tsp caster (superfine) sugar

2.5 ml/½ tsp arrowroot

100 ml/3½ fl oz/scant ½ cup no-fat Greek yoghurt

Sprigs of mint, to decorate

1 Prepare the fruit, reserving a few for decoration, and put in a heavy-based saucepan with the sugar. Cook over a low heat for 2–3 minutes until the fruit is tender.

2 Mix the arrowroot with 10 ml/2 tsp cold water. Add to the fruit and simmer for 1 minute, until thickened. Allow to cool. Spoon two-thirds of the mixture into two glasses.

3 Mash the remaining fruit with a fork and pass through a sieve (strainer) to remove the pips. Fold the fruit purée into the yoghurt.

4 Spoon the yoghurt mixture into the glasses. Chill for 30 minutes before serving decorated with the reserved fruit and small sprigs of mint.

Fresh Raspberry Sorbet

SERVES 4		115 CALORIES PER SERVING

93% CARBOHYDRATE	2% PROTEIN	2% FAT	3% ALCOHOL

100 g/4 oz/½ cup granulated sugar

75 ml/5 tbsp water

15 ml/1 tbsp raspberry or orange liqueur

225 g/8 oz fresh raspberries

15 ml/1 tbsp lemon juice

Small sprigs of mint, to garnish

1 Put the sugar in a pan with the water and heat gently until the sugar dissolves. Bring to the boil and boil for 1 minute. Remove from the heat and allow to cool. Stir in the liqueur.

2 Reserve a few raspberries for decoration. Put the remainder with the lemon juice in a blender or food processor and blend until smooth. Rub the purée through a sieve (strainer) to remove the pips.

3 Blend the raspberry purée and sugar syrup together. Pour into a shallow freezerproof container and freeze for about 4 hours, removing from the freezer every hour and whisking well to break up the ice crystals.

4 Scoop the sorbet into chilled glasses and serve straight away, decorated with a few fresh raspberries and sprigs of mint.

Melon and Ginger Water Ice

SERVES 4	105 CALORIES PER SERVING

88% CARBOHYDRATE	12% PROTEIN	NO FAT

1 honeydew melon

30 ml/2 tbsp caster (superfine) sugar

2.5 ml/½ tsp ground ginger

Juice of 1 lime

2 egg whites

1 Halve the melon, remove the seeds and scoop out the flesh and roughly chop. Put the sugar, ginger and lime juice in a small saucepan and gently heat until the sugar has dissolved. Leave to cool.

2 Put the melon in a food processor with the ginger syrup and blend until smooth. Pour into a freezerproof container and freeze for 2 hours.

3 Whisk the egg whites until stiff, whisk the melon purée, then fold the egg whites into the purée. Return to the container and freeze for at least 2 hours. Scoop into individual chilled dishes to serve.

Frozen Vanilla Yoghurt

SERVES 4		110 CALORIES PER SERVING
65% CARBOHYDRATE	30% PROTEIN	5% FAT

100 ml/3½ fl oz/scant ½ cup skimmed milk

2.5 ml/½ tsp powdered gelatine

400 ml/14 fl oz/1¾ cups no-fat Greek yoghurt

50 g/2 oz/⅛ cup clear honey

5 ml/1 tsp vanilla essence (extract)

1 egg white

Fresh fruit, to serve (optional)

1 Pour 60 ml/4 tbsp milk into a small bowl. Sprinkle over the gelatine. Leave to soak for 5 minutes, then place the bowl over a pan of near-boiling water and stir until dissolved. Cool for 5 minutes, then stir into the rest of the milk.

2 Mix the yoghurt, honey and vanilla essence together, then stir in the milk. Whisk the egg white until soft peaks form, then fold into the yoghurt mixture.

3 Pour the mixture into a freezerproof container and freeze for 2 hours. Remove and beat the mixture to break up the ice crystals. Return to the freezer. Repeat twice more at half-hourly intervals, then freeze until firm.

4 Transfer to the fridge to soften for 20 minutes before serving. Scoop into chilled glasses and serve straight away, with fresh fruit, if liked.

Strawberry and Lemon Filo Tartlets

MAKES 6	70 CALORIES PER SERVING

65% CARBOHYDRATE	8% PROTEIN	27% FAT

3 sheets of filo pastry (paste)

15 g/½ oz/1 tbsp butter or polyunsaturated spread, melted

30 ml/2 tbsp lemon curd

45 ml/3 tbsp no-fat Greek yoghurt

175 g/6 oz small strawberries

15 ml/1 tbsp redcurrant jelly (clear conserve)

1 Cut the pastry into 18 17.5 cm/3 in squares. Layer three squares in each of six sections of a shallow non-stick bun tin (patty pan), overlapping to make a star, and lightly brushing between the layers with butter or spread.

2 Bake the filo pastry cases (shells) in a preheated oven at 190°C/375°F/gas mark 5 for 10 minutes, or until lightly browned and crisp.

3 Put the lemon curd in a small bowl and stir until smooth. Add the Greek yoghurt and mix together. Spoon into the pastry cases.

4 Hull the strawberries and arrange on top of the lemon cream, placing a whole one in the centre and four or five halves around it. Melt the redcurrant jelly and brush over the strawberries to glaze. Serve within 2 hours of filling.

Dark Chocolate Soufflés

SERVES 4	180 CALORIES PER SERVING

58% CARBOHYDRATE	12% PROTEIN	30% FAT

40 g/1½ oz plain (semi-sweet) chocolate

15 ml/1 tbsp cocoa (unsweetened chocolate) powder

10 ml/2 tsp cornflour (cornstarch)

45 ml/3 tbsp caster (superfine) sugar

100 ml/3½ fl oz/scant ½ cup skimmed milk

2 eggs, separated

10 ml/2 tsp icing (confectioners') sugar, to dust

1 Roughly chop the chocolate and put in a non-stick pan with the cocoa powder, cornflour and 10 ml/2 tsp caster sugar. Add a little of the milk and blend to a smooth paste, then stir in the remaining milk.

2 Gradually bring to the boil over a low heat, stirring all the time until the mixture thickens. Remove from the heat and leave until tepid, stirring occasionally. Stir in the egg yolks.

3 Whisk the egg whites until they form soft peaks. Whisk in the remaining caster sugar, 5 ml/1 tsp at a time, until stiff and glossy. Stir one-third into the chocolate mixture, then carefully fold in the remainder.

4 Divide the mixture between four 150 ml/¼ pt/⅔ cup ramekins (custard cups). Put on a hot baking (cookie) sheet in an oven preheated to 190°C/375°F/gas mark 5 for 12 minutes or until well risen. Dust with icing sugar and serve straight away.

Rum-baked Bananas

SERVES 2   235 CALORIES PER SERVING

63% CARBOHYDRATE   5% PROTEIN   25% FAT   7% ALCOHOL

2 large bananas

Finely grated rind and juice of ½ orange

A pinch of ground cinnamon

A pinch of grated nutmeg

15 g/½ oz/1 tbsp butter or polyunsaturated margarine

15 ml/1 tbsp soft light brown sugar

30 ml/2 tbsp dark rum or coconut liqueur

60 ml/4 tbsp plain yoghurt

1 Peel the bananas, thickly slice on the diagonal and arrange in a single layer in a shallow ovenproof dish. Sprinkle with the grated orange rind, cinnamon and nutmeg.

2 Put the orange juice, butter or margarine and sugar in a small pan and heat gently until the sugar has dissolved. Stir in the rum or liqueur. Pour over the bananas.

3 Bake in a preheated oven at 180ºC/350ºF/gas mark 4 for 15 minutes or until golden and bubbling. Serve hot with the yoghurt.

Grilled Papaya with Ginger

SERVES 2		60 CALORIES PER SERVING
94% CARBOHYDRATE	5% PROTEIN	1% FAT

1 papaya

Juice of 1 lime

20 ml/4 tsp caster (superfine) sugar

5 ml/1 tsp ground ginger

1 Cut the papaya in half lengthwise. Scoop out and discard the black seeds. Cut each half lengthwise into four slices. Arrange flesh-side up on a grill (broiler) pan.

2 Sprinkle the lime juice over the papaya. Mix the caster sugar and ground ginger together. Sprinkle over the papaya.

3 Cook under a preheated grill for 3–4 minutes, or until the sugar has caramelised and the fruit is tender. Serve warm.

Baked Amaretti Peaches

SERVES 2		225 CALORIES PER SERVING
62% CARBOHYDRATE	11% PROTEIN	27% FAT

2 large ripe peaches

Finely grated rind and juice of ½ lemon

25 g/1 oz amaretti biscuits

15 g/½ oz/2 tbsp toasted chopped hazelnuts (filberts)

15 ml/1 tbsp soft light brown sugar

10 ml/2 tsp clear honey

45 ml/3 tbsp no-fat Greek yoghurt, to serve

Mint leaves, to decorate

1 Cut the peaches in half and remove the stones (pits). Dip each peach half in the lemon juice, then put in an ovenproof dish.

2 Lightly crush the amaretti biscuits and put in a bowl with the hazelnuts, sugar and lemon rind. Mix together.

3 Divide the mixture between the peaches and press down lightly. Bake in a preheated oven at 180°C/350°F/gas mark 4 for 15 minutes or until the filling is lightly browned.

4 Drizzle over the honey and place two peach halves on each plate with a spoonful of Greek yoghurt. Decorate with fresh mint leaves.

Poached Pears with Fudgy Chocolate Sauce

SERVES 4		195 CALORIES
82% CARBOHYDRATE	6% PROTEIN	12% FAT

4 firm medium pears

30 ml/2 tbsp lemon juice

75 g/3 oz/scant ½ cup golden caster (superfine) sugar

30 ml/2 tbsp golden (light corn) syrup

375 ml/13fl oz/1½ cups water

50 g/2 oz/½ cup cocoa (unsweetened chocolate) powder

5 ml/1 tsp vanilla essence (extract)

1 Peel the pears, leaving them whole with the stalks intact. Using an apple corer or teaspoon, scoop out the core end from the base of each pear. Immediately after peeling, brush the pears with the lemon juice to prevent them from going brown.

2 Put 50 g/2 oz/¼ cup sugar in a heavy-based pan, in which the pears will just fit, with the golden syrup and water. Heat gently until the sugar dissolves, then bring to the boil. Add the pears, cover and simmer for 20 minutes, until the pears are tender. Transfer the pears to a serving dish.

3 Boil the syrup until reduced to 250 ml/8 fl oz/1 cup. Blend the cocoa powder with the remaining sugar and 60 ml/4 tbsp cold water. Stir in a few spoonfuls of the syrup, then whisk the cocoa paste into the remaining syrup in the pan. Bring to the boil and simmer for 2 minutes, stirring constantly.

4 Remove the sauce from the heat, stir in the vanilla essence and leave until warm. Spoon a little of the sauce over the pears and serve the rest separately.

Tip: When poaching, cover the pears with a piece of crumpled greaseproof paper to keep them submerged in the syrup.

Autumn Pudding

SERVES 6		220 CALORIES PER SERVING
89% CARBOHYDRATE	9% PROTEIN	2% FAT

350 g/12 oz cooking (tart) apples, cored and chopped

350 g/12 oz plums, halved, stoned (pitted) and chopped

225 g/8 oz blackberries

50 g/2 oz/¼ cup caster (superfine) sugar

150 ml/¼ pt/⅔ cup cranberry or apple juice

10 slices of thinly-cut day-old white bread

No-fat Greek yoghurt or whipped cream, to serve

1 Put the apples, plums, blackberries, sugar and cranberry or apple juice into a saucepan. Bring to the boil, cover and simmer gently for 10–12 minutes or until the apple is soft. Remove from the heat and leave to cool.

2 Trim the crusts off the bread. Cut a round of bread to fit the base of a 1.5 litre/2½ pt/6 cup pudding basin. Cut the remaining bread into wide strips. Put aside three strips and arrange the rest around the sides of the basin, overlapping them slightly.

3 Reserve 60 ml/4 tbsp fruit juice. Spoon the fruit into the lined bowl, filling almost to the top. Cover with the remaining slices of bread.

4 Put a plate or saucer on top and weigh down. Chill for at least 4 hours, or overnight.

5 Run a knife around the edge of the pudding and turn out on to a serving plate. Brush the reserved juices over any patches of bread that are still white. Cut the pudding into wedges to serve with no-fat Greek yoghurt or whipped cream.

SNACKS AND BAKES

Snacks, cakes and biscuits don't have to be banned altogether from a slimming diet. The occasional nibble between meals can help control appetite and help you to stick to the diet. The trouble is, when hunger pangs strike, you don't just feel 'a bit peckish': a slice of gooey chocolate cake is always much more desirable than a low-fat yoghurt or crispbread.

To solve the problem, this chapter is full of delicious but healthy low-calorie bakes, including Date and Oat Slices (page 146) and Chocolate and Cherry Sponge (page 152). They're ideal for social occasions when you want to join in without over-indulging. Ideally, freeze these treats in individual portions but if you know you won't be able to stop at one slice, then give them a miss altogether.

Remember that snacks are not a compulsary part of the diet! If you're not hungry, leave them out and have a piece of fresh fruit instead.

Bruschetta with Goats' Cheese, Rocket and Sun-dried Tomato

SERVES 2		195 CALORIES PER SERVING
52% CARBOHYDRATE	18% PROTEIN	30% FAT

4 medium slices from a country-style loaf

1 garlic clove

10 ml/2 tsp olive oil

50 g/2 oz/¼ cup soft goats' cheese

4 sun-dried tomatoes in oil, drained

Rocket leaves

Salt and freshly ground black pepper

1 Put the bread on a grill (broiler) pan and grill (broil) under a low heat for 3–4 minutes, until dry and just beginning to colour. Turn over and grill the other side.

2 Cut the garlic clove in half, rub the cut surfaces over the bread and brush with the olive oil.

3 Spread the cheese thickly over the bruschetta. Pat excess oil from the tomatoes with kitchen paper (paper towels), then chop and arrange them on top of the cheese, with a few rocket leaves.

4 Lightly season with salt and ground pepper. Serve as soon as possible after topping.

Alternative Toppings

Hummus and Olives: Thickly spread 75 g/3 oz reduced-fat hummus over the bruschetta. Roughly chop 10 black olives in brine and scatter over the hummus.

Smoked Salmon and Horseradish: Mix 30 ml/2 tbsp half-fat crème fraîche, 5 ml/1 tsp creamed horseradish and 15 ml/1 tbsp chopped fresh dill (dill weed) together and spread over the bruschetta. Snip 40 g/1½ oz smoked salmon into small pieces and arrange on top. Garnish with sprigs of dill.

Blue Cheese and Chives: Crumble 40 g/1½ oz blue cheese and scatter over the bruschetta. Just before serving, grill (broil) for 1 minute until the cheese just begins to melt. Sprinkle with 15 ml/1 tbsp snipped fresh chives.

Feta Cheese Scones

MAKES 10		90 CALORIES PER SCONE
63% CARBOHYDRATE	18% PROTEIN	19% FAT

100 g/4 oz/1 cup self-raising (self-rising) flour

100 g/4 oz/1 cup self-raising wholemeal flour

2.5 ml/½ tsp salt

75 g/3 oz/scant ½ cup Feta cheese

150 ml/¼ pt/⅔ cup skimmed milk, plus extra for glazing

1.5 ml/¼ tsp paprika (optional)

1 Sift the flours and salt into a mixing bowl, adding the bran left in the sieve (strainer). Crumble the Feta cheese and rub into the dry ingredients.

2 Make a well in the middle, add the milk and mix to a soft dough. Turn out on to a lightly floured surface and knead for a few seconds until smooth.

3 Roll out the dough to about 2 cm/¾ in thick and stamp out scones (biscuits) using a 6 cm/2½ in biscuit (cookie) cutter. Place on a non-stick baking (cookie) sheet. Brush the tops with a little skimmed milk and sprinkle with paprika, if liked.

4 Bake in a preheated oven at 200°C/400°F/gas mark 6 for 15 minutes, or until golden brown. Cool on a wire rack and serve warm or cold with a scraping of low-fat spread.

Tip: For a sweet version, add 15 ml/1 tbsp caster (superfine) sugar to the flours when making the scones, omit the paprika and serve with reduced-sugar jam (conserve).

Summer Fruit Platter with Crushed Cantucci

SERVES 1		105 CALORIES PER SERVING
67% CARBOHYDRATE	8% PROTEIN	25% FAT

225 g/8 oz fresh fruit, eg strawberries, raspberries, cherries, peaches or apricots

50 g/2 oz cantucci biscuits

1 Wash and prepare the fruit, cutting the larger fruit into halves or slices. Arrange on a platter.

2 Roughly chop or crush the cantucci with a rolling pin and scatter over the fruit. Serve within an hour of making.

Date and Oat Slices

MAKES 8   230 CALORIES PER SLICE

65% CARBOHYDRATE   6% PROTEIN   29% FAT

175 g/6 oz/¾ cup dried stoned (pitted) dates

150 ml/¼ pt/⅔ cup orange juice

2.5 ml/½ tsp ground ginger

100 g/4 oz/1 cup plain (all-purpose) flour

2.5 ml/½ tsp ground cinnamon

2.5 ml/½ tsp baking powder

1.5 ml/¼ tsp bicarbonate of soda (baking soda)

A pinch of salt

65 g/2½ oz/scant ⅓ cup butter or polyunsaturated spread

50 g/2 oz/¼ cup soft light brown sugar

75 g/3 oz/¾ cup rolled oats

1 Roughly chop the dates and put in a small saucepan with the orange juice and ginger. Slowly bring to the boil and simmer for 10 minutes, or until the dates are softened. Mash to a smooth purée. Leave to cool.

2 Sift the flour, cinnamon, baking powder, bicarbonate of soda and salt into a mixing bowl. Rub in the butter or spread until the mixture resembles breadcrumbs. Stir in the sugar and oats.

3 Press half the crumb mixture firmly into a 20 cm/8 in square baking tin (pan). Spoon in the date mixture, spreading out evenly. Sprinkle over the remaining crumb mixture and press down lightly.

4 Bake in a preheated oven at 160°C/325°F/gas mark 3 for 25–30 minutes or until lightly browned. Cool in the tin, then cut into eight fingers to serve.

Greek Yoghurt with Fresh Dates and Almonds

SERVES 2		235 CALORIES PER SERVING
49% CARBOHYDRATE	21% PROTEIN	30% FAT

100 g/4 oz fresh dates

200 g/7 oz/1 small carton of no-fat Greek yoghurt

25 g/1 oz/¼ cup unskinned almonds

30 ml/2 tbsp clear honey

1 Stone (pit) the dates and roughly chop. Chop the almonds. Put a few chopped dates and almonds in the bottom of two glass dishes, then spoon in half the yoghurt.

2 Top with the remaining dates and yoghurt. Scatter with the rest of the chopped almonds, then drizzle over the honey.

Three-bean Tahini Dip with Breadsticks and Crudités

SERVES 4		235 CALORIES PER SERVING
54% CARBOHYDRATES	21% PROTEIN	25% FAT

200 g/7 oz/1 small can of borlotti beans

200 g/7 oz/1 small can of cannellini beans

200 g/7 oz/1 small can of flageolet beans

1 garlic clove, peeled and crushed

Juice of 1 lemon

30 ml/2 tbsp tahini paste

30 ml/2 tbsp boiling water

15 ml/1 tbsp chopped fresh parsley

Salt and freshly ground black pepper

2 medium carrots

2 celery sticks

8 breadsticks

1 Drain all the beans, rinse under cold water, then drain again. Put in a blender or food processor with the garlic, lemon juice and tahini. Blend until smooth.

2 Add the boiling water, parsley, salt and pepper and blend again until very smooth. Taste and add a little more seasoning, if needed. Spoon into a serving bowl, cover and chill until ready to serve.

3 Prepare the carrots and celery and cut into 7.5 cm/3 in sticks. Serve the dip on a plate surrounded by the carrots and celery and breadsticks.

Fruit and Nut Crunch Bars

MAKES 12		100 CALORIES PER SLICE
62% CARBOHYDRATE	8% PROTEIN	30% FAT

250 g/9 oz/1½ cups dried fruit salad, roughly chopped

75 g/3 oz/½ cup raisins

30 ml/2 tbsp orange juice

30 ml/2 tbsp clear honey

25 g/1 oz/¼ cup chopped mixed nuts

30 ml/2 tbsp sesame seeds

30 ml/2 tbsp pumpkin seeds

25 g/1 oz/½ cup puffed rice cereal

1 Put the fruit salad, raisins, orange juice and honey in a food processor and process until fairly smooth. Add the nuts, sesame seeds and pumpkin seeds and process for a few more seconds.

2 Tip the mixture into a bowl and stir in the puffed rice cereal. Spoon into a shallow 20 cm/8 in tin (pan), lined with non-stick baking parchment, smoothing the top with the back of a spoon.

3 Chill in the fridge for 2 hours, then cut into 12 slices. Remove from the tin and store in an airtight container.

Spiced Yoghurt Cake

SERVES 12		160 CALORIES PER SLICE
78% CARBOHYDRATE	10% PROTEIN	12% FAT

5 ml/1 tsp bicarbonate of soda (baking soda)

250 ml/8 fl oz/1 cup no-fat Greek yoghurt

40 g/1½ oz/3 tbsp butter or sunflower margarine

175 g/6 oz/¾ cup light soft brown sugar

5 ml/1 tsp vanilla essence (extract)

1 egg, beaten

225 g/8 oz/2 cups plain (all-purpose) flour

10 ml/2 tsp baking powder

5 ml/1 tsp ground cinnamon

2.5 ml/½ tsp ground ginger

1 Blend the bicarbonate of soda with a little yoghurt in a large jug or bowl. Stir in the remaining yoghurt and set aside for 5 minutes – the mixture will froth up.

2 Put the butter or margarine, sugar, vanilla essence and half the egg in a bowl. Beat together until light and creamy, then gradually mix in the rest of the egg.

3 Sift the flour, baking powder and spices together. Fold into the mixture with the yoghurt. Spoon into a 20 cm/8 in square cake tin (pan), lined with non-stick baking paper.

4 Bake on the middle shelf of a preheated oven at 180°C/350°F/gas mark 4 for 35–40 minutes, or until a skewer inserted into the middle of the cake comes out clean.

5 Allow the cake to cool in the tin for 10 minutes, then turn out on a cooling rack. When completely cold, cut into 12 slices.

Tip: This cake is equally good served warm as a dessert. Accompany with low-fat custard or plain yoghurt.

Chocolate and Cherry Sponge

No one will guess that this cake contains prunes. When puréed with a little water, they can be used instead of butter to give cakes a rich moist texture.

MAKES 8 SLICES		265 CALORIES PER SLICE
79% CARBOHYDRATE	9% PROTEIN	12% FAT

75 g/3 oz/½ cup stoned (pitted) dried prunes

30 ml/2 tbsp water

175 g/6 oz/¾ cup soft light brown sugar

3 eggs

150 g/5 oz/1¼ cups self-raising (self-rising) flour

25 g/1 oz/¼ cup cocoa (unsweetened chocolate) powder

2.5 ml/½ tsp baking powder

75 g/3 oz/½ cup dried cherries

75 g/3 oz/generous ¼ cup black cherry jam (conserve)

15 ml/1 tbsp icing (confectioners') sugar, to dust

1 Put the prunes in a food processor with 30 ml/2 tbsp cold water and blend to a smooth purée. Transfer to a mixing bowl. Add the soft brown sugar and eggs and whisk until thick and foamy.

2 Sift the flour, cocoa powder and baking powder into the bowl and carefully fold in with the cherries.

3 Divide the mixture between two 18 cm/7 in non-stick sandwich tins (pans), base-lined with non-stick baking parchment.

4 Bake in a preheated oven at 180°C/350°F/gas mark 4 for 15 minutes, until the sponges are well-risen and springy to the touch.

5 Turn the sponges out on to a wire rack to cool. When cold, sandwich together with black cherry jam and dust the top with icing sugar.

Carrot and Courgette Cake with Cream Cheese Frosting

MAKES 10 SLICES		115 CALORIES PER SLICE
53% CARBOHYDRATE	17% PROTEIN	30% FAT

1 medium carrot, peeled

1 medium courgette (zucchini)

100 g/4 oz/½ cup soft light brown sugar

3 eggs, separated

Finely grated rind of 1 orange

75 g/3 oz/¾ cup self-raising (self-rising) flour

50 g/2 oz/½ cup self-raising wholemeal flour

5 ml/1 tsp ground mixed (apple-pie) spice

For the Cream Cheese Frosting:

150 g/5 oz/scant ¾ cup low-fat soft cheese

15 g/½ oz icing (confectioners') sugar, sifted

5 ml/1 tsp vanilla essence (extract)

1 Coarsely grate the carrot and the courgette.

2 Put the sugar, egg yolks and orange rind in a bowl and whisk until very thick and light.

3 Sift the flours and mixed spice over the whisked mixture, adding the bran left in the sieve (strainer) and fold in together with the grated vegetables.

4 Whisk the egg whites until stiff but not dry. Stir a third into the mixture, then carefully fold in the rest. Spoon into a base-lined and greased 18 cm/7 in square cake tin (pan) and level the top.

5 Bake in a preheated oven at 180°C/350°F/gas mark 4 for 55 minutes, covering with foil if the top starts to brown too much. Cool in the tin for 10 minutes, then turn out and cool on a wire rack.

6 For the frosting, beat together the cheese, icing sugar and vanilla essence. Spread over the cake, roughening the surface with a palette knife. Keep chilled in the fridge until ready to serve.

INDEX